Scars of Gold

A Midwife's personal story of birth trauma and recovery

Sharon Stoliar

Scars of Gold

hello@sharonstoliar.com
www.sharonstoliar.com

ISBN: 978-1-922854-70-4 (Paperback)
978-1-922854-71-1 (eBook)

NATIONAL LIBRARY OF AUSTRALIA
A catalogue record for this book is available from the National Library of Australia

Editors: Jason Martin and Chloe Cran
Cover Design: Ocean Reeve Publishing
Design and Typeset: Ocean Reeve Publishing
Printed in Australia by Ocean Reeve Publishing

Published by Sharon Stoliar and Ocean Reeve Publishing
www.oceanreevepublishing.com

Ocean REEVE PUBLISHING

Endorsements for Scars of Gold

"The healthcare system can be an impersonal and unforgiving place, but the people who work in it can find themselves in the role of patients as well as caregivers. They are therefore subject to the same issues and challenges as others in the community, but have a unique perspective spanning both sides of the clinical relationship.

By sharing her personal experiences, Sharon Stoliar highlights how difficult it can be to be heard in healthcare, and the devastating impact it can have on the health and future of affected individuals. She also highlights the simple things that make a difference but are often overlooked, and from this offers a roadmap to better outcomes.

This book should be required reading for all healthcare practitioners and students, and will improve the quality of care they provide. I am delighted to recommend it."

Professor Vlado Perkovic
Dean of Medicine and Scientia Professor,
University of New South Wales

"Sharon Stoliar is the epitome of what it means to be hero. Where most would run from painful memories, Sharon holds hers close, using her brave voice to demand change for the rest of us."

Amber Petty
Author, Mental Health Ambassador, Foster Carer,
Host of The Wise Guides

"Sharon's story is shocking, but one that is all too common. By shedding light on the widespread reality of birth trauma Sharon will empower women to have safer, healthier births. Valuable research and an enriching read for mums-to-be and the nursing, birthing, and medical staff who support them."

Dr Justin Coulson

Best Selling Author, co-host & parenting expert of Channel 9's Parental Guidance, Psychologist

This is a wonderful book tackling birth and trauma in a compassionate and thoughtful way. Sharon gives voice to many of the themes women and partners feel after a traumatic perinatal period. It's so important we hear these stories and narratives of birth and healing.

Dr Rebecca Moore

Perinatal Psychiatrist & Make Birth Better co-founder

After all these years, it remains a searing tragedy, that we are still not getting birthing right. That in our modern world, with all our scientific advances, something so basic goes wrong at a human level for so many mothers and their partners. Sharon Stoliar writes as both a midwife, and a person who has experienced severe outcomes from birthing herself. And who identifies the core problem in a way that can be fixed. We have to prioritize deep listening and respect for the mother at birth. We have to make midwives and doctors' lives workable so they can afford the time to do this. Otherwise the echoes of trauma for mother, baby, and health carer will continue to do immense harm, as they have for centuries. We need to fix this now. This book is an unforgettable signpost to how we do that.

Steve Biddulph AM

Best Selling Author, Activist, Psychologist

"Birth Trauma is real. Birth Trauma experienced at the hands of care providers is also very real.

Reading Sharon's painful and incredibly personal story is yet another insight into what is happening within our maternity care system. #ItsTime to return to kindness, compassion, empathy and really listening to women/people - as the compulsory prerequisite for ALL birthing women/people."

Zoe Naylor
Producer, Activist, co-founder of the Birth Time movement,
co-writer, director & producer of Birth Time: the documentary

"The miracle of birth, is just that. A miracle. If everyone makes it out of there okay, we say, that's all that matters. And of course, in the big picture, there's truth to that. Yet, research tells us, birth experiences matter a great deal when it comes to how things unfold in those first few months of a child's life. And unfortunately, in many cases- can have a negative impact for years. In Scars of Gold, Sharon's post labour experience depicts the physical and emotional damage, that can occur when women aren't listened to. Sharon's story exposes the raw pain of a traumatic birth, and the hope that her experience would change the way maternity care is provided to women."

Ally Barnes
Radio Presenter & Producer, Hope 103.2

"Sharon's story is a moving personal account of the damage birth trauma can inflict on new, vulnerable mums. She is truly brave for laying it all bare so that others may learn from her experience. Left with crippling injuries and battling a sea of emotions for many years, Sharon is fighting to speak her truth and to have birth trauma recognised.

I fought back tears as I read each page feeling every emotion Sharon endured. It's a compelling read that will leave you with many questions about how we can get it so wrong in this day and age."

Chezzi Denyer

Senior TV Produce, Creative Director, & Presenter - Mummy Time TV

Sharon's reflections hit me far more personally than anticipated, due to a non-obstetric incident where a hospital 'accidentally' overdosed me, finding my blue-black body lying dead in my own vomit, so many of Sharon's comments hit that raw nerve "...bitterly betrayed by the healthcare system I had placed all of my faith in ... I was one of their own, but they had utterly let me down ... [with their] lack of proper care ... the system that used me, chewed me up, and unceremoniously spat me out ... I received a copy of my records ... Each entry I read through left me more furious than the one before ... To say I was angry at what I was reading was an understatement. I was enraged."

And as a woman who has given birth several times, I became a Midwife who strongly advocated throughout my career, to passionately prevent avoidable birth trauma, and to thoroughly debrief unavoidable birth trauma, because I know how dreadfully it can haunt a mother, for the rest of her life. Sharon gives sound to the many unheard voices."

Kathy Fray

Midwife & Best-selling Maternity Author

"Sharon's powerful story highlights how important it is for a woman to be heard during her birth and recovery and how we as medical professionals can be both the answer and the problem in our patient's care.

This experience can help so many women find their voice but also be a wakeup call to doctors and other health professionals about being dismissive."

Dr Jana Pittman
Mother, Wife, Doctor, World Champion, Olympian

Thank you to Sharon Stoliar for bravely and transparently telling her story of birth-related trauma. While complications may be missed or incorrectly diagnosed even in the best medical systems, Sharon describes the real source of trauma: not being heard, seen, or believed. Her account reminds us of the most fundamental care principal. Namely, that the people we serve are experts in their own experiences and bodies and it is our duty to learn from what they tell us, to approach our care with empathy and humility, and to fully embrace their position at the center of the care team.

Dr Joan Combellick PHD MPH CNM FACNM
Assistant Professor
Co-Specialty Director, Midwifery
Yale School of Nursing

Disclaimer

Names and identifying features have been changed to protect the identities of certain individuals.

Dedication

For my family, for holding me up when I couldn't hold myself.

For Sally, for being my advocate and my voice when I lost my own.

For Ronen, for holding my hand and walking beside me every day.

For Jeremy, for being my lifeline and my source of joy when my world was dark.

For my Jehovah-Rapha, you are the God that heals.

And for every mother who has suffered birth trauma. May this book bring you hope for healing and encouragement to find your voice to speak up.

Preface

A few years ago, I was asked to share my story at a maternity care conference at one of the local health districts in Sydney.

On 17 March 2017, I shared my birth story for the first time in a public forum. I thought it would be easy because, at that time, it had been over five years and I had written so much about it for clinical purposes, but it was probably the hardest and most emotional speech I'll ever give in my life. I spoke about my own birth experience and the importance of healthcare workers' attitudes, and the importance of listening to women in the context of maternity care services. I spoke about birth trauma and the cost of not listening to women. When I stood up there and saw an auditorium full of midwives staring at me, I nearly ran out of the room before I opened my mouth. And yet, I knew God had placed me there for a reason, and it was only by His grace and strength that I stood there and spoke the words that I had written down. And it was that day—when I had the courage to look up in between words and saw the faces of the midwives, quietly listening with tears streaming down some of their faces—that I finally realised the power of sharing my story.

I became a mum in November 2011. Within twenty-four hours of giving birth, I developed acute compartment syndrome in my right lower leg. Acute compartment syndrome is a rare complication in the postpartum period, but it requires urgent decompressive surgery (a fasciotomy) to prevent permanent damage and amputation. Mine was not diagnosed definitively until day ten, although it had been suspected by a neurologist at a much earlier stage.

It's been almost ten years now, and you can't tell that I live with physical pain every single day.

Each step I take hurts. It hurts to drive for more than an hour. It hurts to stand for more than thirty minutes. For a long time, it hurt to jump and run and do all the fun, crazy things that kids like to do with their mammas. It still does hurt to run around and play.

Over the years, my left side has learned to carry more of my weight and compensate really well for the weaknesses in my right side. As a result, the muscles in my right leg remain weak unless I continue with strict exercises and physiotherapy to stop the muscles wasting away any more than they already have. My orthopaedic surgeon says that I will likely have to work at keeping my right side strong for the rest of my life; otherwise, my ability to keep my balance will deteriorate. However, I am amazed at how remarkable my recovery has been. While there are deficits, it is quite miraculous just how well I can walk now, considering I could have lost my leg.

But every single time I feel the pain, I know it is nothing short of a miracle that I still have a leg to feel the pain in. The doctors said it was because I had age on my side, and my peripheral circulation was so good that it kept my leg alive. I am thankful to God that I still have my leg, that I can still walk and look after my son and live my life.

I am at peace with my life now, but I didn't always feel this way. I was angry for a long time. I was angry at the hospital. Angry at the doctors and midwives who refused to listen to me and *see* the physical pain I was in while I was complaining to them about the agonising pain in my leg. I wanted them to see just how much this has impacted my life and those close to me.

Nothing could have prevented the compartment syndrome from developing, but listening to me could have significantly changed the outcome. I often thought that maybe if they listened to me, I could have had the surgery I needed, and I wouldn't have the physical restrictions and pain that I have now. Maybe.

Prologue

'You have acute compartment syndrome,' I heard. It was two o'clock in the morning. Maybe I was in the middle of a nightmare.

'What?' I asked.

The doctor replied, 'You have acute compartment syndrome; the surgical team will see you in the morning.'

I couldn't understand this. Her cheery voice contradicted the gravity of the diagnosis being delivered to me. My head was spinning. My nursing training kicked in. *Isn't compartment syndrome an emergency? Shouldn't they be whisking me off into theatres like in so many scenes I'd watched in* Grey's Anatomy *or* ER? *Like in real-life situations I had been involved in?* I had never seen acute compartment syndrome in my short-lived nursing and midwifery career, but I knew from way back in my undergraduate university days that ACS is a medical emergency and I should be rushed off to theatres now!

My train of thought was suddenly interrupted. 'You're nurse-trained, aren't you?'

'Yes,' I replied, in disbelief that she was even making me refer to my clinical knowledge at a time like this.

'You'll know more about it than me, but you can talk about it with the surgeons in the morning.'

She didn't give me time to ask any more questions. I had been waiting all day to get my MRI results. Each time I asked the midwives, they awkwardly changed the subject and said they would get someone to come in and discuss the findings with me. I had worked as a midwife and looked after hundreds of postnatal women. I knew something wasn't right. I had seen many things go wrong in the postnatal ward, but I also knew what was normal. Nothing about my right leg was normal, and nothing about the way the midwives were evading my questions about my MRI result was normal.

Before the MRI, they told me it would be a quick twenty-minute scan because they didn't *really* believe the neurologists' earlier suspicions of acute compartment syndrome. The MRI had taken much longer than they prepared me for. The doctors kept dismissing it because they had 'never seen it in obstetrics, so it couldn't possibly be compartment syndrome'. But alas, it was. After being told repeatedly that it couldn't be compartment syndrome, in the dead of night, a registrar came and delivered the very diagnosis they said it couldn't be.

Such a brief interaction to be delivered such a scary diagnosis. A myriad of thoughts and fears were spinning through my head; I wasn't thinking clinically. I couldn't. I was in pain. I couldn't reach into the crevice of my clinical brain to think as a midwife, not with the agony, and not with the new baby hormones surging through my body, taking away all my ability to control my emotions. I asked her, 'Is my leg going to burst open before they see me?' And she replied, in her cheery, chirpy, singsong voice, 'I sure hope not,' as if I had just asked her if it was going to rain today.

And with that, she was gone.

Instead of being a low-risk childbearing woman, I had suddenly become a sick 'patient', along with all the connotations that go with being that.

'What's compartment syndrome?' I heard, my mum's shaky voice breaking through the silence. I didn't know how to answer her. The tears were uncontrollable. I couldn't speak. I googled ACS on my phone and handed it to her to read the Wikipedia.

I never appreciated just how scary it must have been for my parents, seeing their adult firstborn on a hospital bed with something crazy happening to her leg, in pain, and the doctors not knowing what is going on. I had no idea just what they must have been feeling through all of this.

Over the years, I have learned that acute compartment syndrome, or ACS, is a limb- and life-threatening medical emergency that requires an urgent fasciotomy to save the affected limb. Without a fasciotomy, ACS can crush the muscles and nerve structures, occluding blood flow, causing significant muscle death and potential permanent disability, which can often require amputation.[1]

---

1 Guo, J., Yin, Y., Jin, L., Zhang, R., Hou, Z., & Zhang, Y. (2019). Acute compartment syndrome: Cause, diagnosis, and new viewpoint. *Medicine, 98*(27), e16260-e16260. doi:10.1097/MD.0000000000016260; McMillan, T. E., Gardner, W. T., Schmidt, A. H., & Johnstone, A. J. (2019). Diagnosing acute compartment syndrome—where have we got to? *International Orthopaedics*, 43(11), 2429-2435. doi:10.1007/s00264-019-04386-y

It was a torturous eight hours, both physically and mentally. *Will I lose my leg?*

I was left to sit with that diagnosis alone, fearing what might happen to my leg between then and the following morning.

Chapter 1

I had a non-eventful and low-risk pregnancy, aside from a short episode of threatened premature labour at twenty-one weeks gestation. After that little scare, I decided it best to take early maternity leave from working twelve-hour shifts in a busy postnatal ward.

When I finally reached term and my waters broke, I was ready. My body worked hard to give birth to this baby, but with a posterior-facing baby, it wasn't an easy feat. I managed to dilate up to seven centimetres before the world of obstetrics deemed me a 'failure to progress' and sent me off to the operating theatre for an emergency caesarean section.

I had planned to push my baby out and go home after four hours. *But, never mind,* I thought. Sometimes a caesarean section is necessary, and this was one of those times. I could accept that, but I would do whatever I could to get out of this hospital as fast as possible. Being a midwife, I knew the best thing for recovery after a caesarean was to get up and move around as much as possible, so the morning after my caesarean, I asked the kind and caring midwife who had been assigned to look after me to help me out of bed as soon as she had time.

After disconnecting my IV lines, she helped me get up and walk to the shower. How wonderful it was to feel the warm water washing away the orange stains of betadine from my skin. I can't remember how long I basked in the bliss of freedom from those wretched IV lines before the unwelcomed pain disrupted my reverie.

I called for my midwife, who promptly came and helped me back to the bed. I can still see the sheen of terror on her face when she saw how red and swollen my leg had become. Being registered nurses as well as midwives, our nursing education kicked in for both of us. What could this be? This was *not* normal. Some swelling in the legs after a caesarean is expected, but *this* wasn't. My right leg had a shiny, red glow to it and was markedly more swollen than my left leg.

My midwife called the doctors to come and review my leg.

After what felt like forever, around two o'clock in the afternoon, a junior resident doctor finally came to see me. By then, my pain levels had significantly increased since the morning shower. She assessed my leg and concluded, 'You must have bumped it in labour. Many women do.'

'But I didn't bump my leg,' I denied, pleading with her for an explanation for this agony.

'You must have knocked it on the bed rail while you were in labour or while you were being taken to the operating theatre,' she insisted.

I knew I hadn't, but it didn't seem to matter to her that I repeatedly denied bumping my leg. She had simply made up her mind to dismiss me. The manner and tone in which she spoke oozed an air of superiority, as if to tell me, 'I'm the doctor and I know more than you, so just be quiet and I'll diagnose you.' She ceremoniously declared my red, swollen, and painful leg to be a muscular injury caused by 'knocking it against the bed rail'.

This doctor knew I was a midwife. *Surely she will respect my own assessment of my pain levels,* I thought. Surely being a midwife meant I had *some* credibility in my assessment of my own body!

This doctor concluded by recommending all the usual things: pain relief, mobilising more, elevating my legs, using a heat pack, and putting some compression stockings on.

As soon as the doctor left the room, I blurted out to my mum, who was in the room with me, 'That doctor doesn't know what she's doing.' I had looked after many women who had caesareans, and I *knew* the swelling in my right leg was not normal.

Later that day, when I was visited by the midwife who looked after me in labour, I asked her if I *had* bumped my leg. Someone was always with me during labour. Between my mum, my sister, my husband, and the midwife, I had never been left alone in the labour room, but I'd begun to second-guess myself after the doctor had insisted upon it. When my midwife and my mother both reinforced what I knew to be true, that I *hadn't* bumped my leg, my frustration grew.

As short-lived as my midwifery career may have been, my training and experience screamed, 'This is not normal. Do something!' But at the same time, I was also very aware that if I voiced my concerns out loud, I'd be labelled as 'the troublemaking know-it-all'.

I felt trapped. Trapped somewhere between being a patient and midwife, afraid of making a fuss but also afraid of the looming disaster in my leg.

As the afternoon progressed, my pain worsened, and I became increasingly distressed. A different obstetric doctor came at eight o'clock in the evening for a routine assessment of the caesarean wound, but she didn't look at my leg, despite me telling her it was worsening. Nothing was done about my leg.

Throughout the rest of the evening, I was 'looked after' by a midwife who made it very clear to me that I was just another bed number on her handover list. I could sense that I frustrated her when I kept pressing the patient buzzer numerous times to complain of my increasing pain levels. I hated pressing that buzzer, but I couldn't do anything for myself.

I felt that she expected me, especially because I was a midwife, to just get on with it and not complain. And believe me, that was *all* I wanted to do. A busy, noisy postnatal ward was *not* where I wanted to be after having my baby. This was not a place where I wanted to experience the transition into motherhood. It was a workplace for me.

My only birth plan had been to push my baby out and go home within four hours. That was all I wanted. I wanted to go home. Why didn't she understand that?

Why was she treating me as if I was being a difficult patient on purpose?

My ability to walk and bear weight continued to deteriorate. Even though I pointed that out to her, she didn't seem to be doing anything about it. She would answer the buzzer in exasperation, roll her eyes, and ask, 'What do you need now?' I could tell she wasn't taking me seriously, and her body language exuded annoyance at having to deal with me.

It suddenly dawned on me that in that patient bed, while I wasn't wearing my work uniform, I was powerless to make them do anything to alleviate my pain. I'd always had this false sense of security in thinking that if I was in hospital, I'd be okay; that if anything were to go wrong, the doctors and midwives around would know what to do.

I had laboured so long and so hard, and all I wanted to do was to get up, carry my gorgeous baby, walk around with him, and actually look after him. I wanted to be the one who was rocking him in my arms and changing his nappies and doing things for him. But there I was, in a hospital bed, unable to get out of bed and walk because of the pain. I couldn't get up and mobilise, as they had told me to, because of the pain. I needed more pain relief, but the pain relief wasn't working. I needed the midwife to pick up my son when he cried and pass him to me. I had to press the buzzer for that, but I could tell it was a nuisance for her.

I asked for my oxycodone (Endone), and that midwife gave me a lecture about looking after my kidneys! Five milligrams of oxycodone! It was nothing! It's not like I was addicted to it. I was in agony—couldn't she see? I demanded to look at my medication chart, which clearly had written on it 'oxycodone PRN', which means as required. Angrily, I said, 'This chart says "Endone PRN". It's now required, so you can go and get me my Endone, thanks!' She wasn't impressed with me, but I was beyond the point of caring what she thought of me.

The oxycodone didn't do anything for the worsening pain. When the first doctor saw me and declared a muscular injury, I was still able to stand up and weight bear. By nine o'clock at night, I couldn't weight bear any longer. The swelling had worsened, I had burning pain down the front of my leg, and the skin was tight and had turned a shiny red colour. I told the midwife who was 'looking after me' that I could no longer bear weight, but for some reason out of this world, she obviously didn't believe I was seriously in pain. Even her documentation in my medical records read with an undertone of disbelief that I was in pain.

By the time the night-shift midwife had started and introduced herself to me, the pain in my leg became so bad that I needed to have more oxycodone. After years of having primary dysmenorrhoea—extremely painful periods—I had a high pain threshold. I didn't even need pain relief for the caesarean; it didn't hurt at all. But this pain was something extraordinary. The night-shift midwife gave me the oxycodone, but again, it didn't do anything to lessen the pain.

That night, the pain gradually increased to a point where I needed to pull the anti-embolism stocking off, which they had put on after the junior doctor instructed earlier that afternoon. My mum was in the room with me and helped me take it off.

My leg instantly ballooned right in front of my eyes.

I felt acute and intense pain, significantly worse than it had been over the afternoon. By this stage, I had started to cry in agony.

It was the most excruciating, agonising pain I had ever felt in my life. At least with labour, I got a break between contractions. But this wasn't like that. It was constant. Unrelenting. Not even a second to breathe.

I thought I was going to die.

I pressed the buzzer, and the midwife came. She tried several things to relieve the pain—repositioning my leg with a pillow under it, elevating it, using a heat pack, an ice pack. Nothing worked. Nothing would alleviate the pain.

It was a harrowing pain that I wouldn't wish on my worst enemy. If I had a knife with me, I would have absolutely cut my leg off. I just wanted my leg gone.

I was crying. My foot had curved inwards—I had foot drop. I couldn't move it. I couldn't wriggle my toes or move my ankle. I couldn't lift my leg up. I couldn't let the midwife touch it. It was raging red and swollen like I'd never seen swelling before.

I didn't know what was happening to me, and I was petrified. I just wanted the pain to go away.

The doctor came to see me. She tried to assess the movement in my leg, but because of the pain, she couldn't touch my leg. Each time she tried, I screamed in agony. She had no idea what it was, but because my usually brown-skinned leg had turned a raging red colour, she suspected I had developed cellulitis.

She inserted a cannula into the back of my hand, collected some bloods for testing, started me on antibiotics, and ordered a 7.5 mg dose of subcutaneous morphine, which the midwife immediately gave me.

After fifteen minutes of having the morphine, my pain remained unchanged. Even an hour later, when I told the midwife through tears that I was still in pain, the midwife told me that the doctor wanted me to 'wait longer to give the morphine more time to work'.

I couldn't understand why they weren't doing anything, why they weren't listening. Wasn't morphine supposed to work sooner than this? Somewhere in my clinical brain, I knew that morphine should work sooner, but in that moment of extreme agony, I just couldn't articulate it. I couldn't think straight to question it. Didn't they believe the agony I was in? It's not like I was making it up. There was something visibly serious going on.

I had to wait until the following morning before anything else was done for me. The doctors came back to tell me that my liver function tests from the blood collected were completely deranged. They determined it to be caused by the antibiotics that I had commenced the previous night, so they changed my antibiotics.

When I think about it now, the doctor had collected my bloods *before* I was given my first dose of antibiotics, which means my liver function was all over the place already, and nobody realised this.

Over the next two days, my neurological symptoms hadn't changed, and although the swelling had slightly improved and the pain wasn't as intensely acute, it was still really painful, and I couldn't get up out of bed. The neurologist, a visiting medical officer, came to see me and said, 'I think you have an acute compartment syndrome. You should have an MRI.'

From then on, there were teams of doctors and midwives coming in and out of my room, but I didn't have that MRI. I don't think that little hospital maternity unit had ever seen so many different teams come to see one patient within days. There was so much back and forth between teams about whether it was or wasn't compartment syndrome. No-one seemed to be able to make up their mind as to whether it was or wasn't compartment syndrome, but somewhere in the back of my head, I knew this was urgent but couldn't really process why they were taking so long to decide if it was. There were too many new mum hormones raging through me at that time, and I couldn't clearly think with my midwife brain.

The surgical consultant said to me, 'I've never seen it in someone who had just had a baby. It can't possibly be compartment syndrome. It has to be cellulitis.'

My antibiotics were changed several times because of liver function tests that continued to be deranged, but my body wasn't responding to any of them. I became a pin cushion, needing a new cannula almost daily because my poor veins kept collapsing with the antibiotics.

Throughout those days, there was a lot of googling, with family members looking up what compartment syndrome is and people telling me that my symptoms sounded like it.

Every time I questioned the doctors, I was always told, 'It's just a query compartment syndrome, but no-one has ever seen it before, so it can't be compartment syndrome.'

I couldn't understand why they were insistent on putting me in the box of 'a mother with a new baby' and couldn't see beyond that. I wasn't just a new mum.

I was actually a surgical patient who had just had major abdominal surgery, and nobody seemed able to see me in this context.

When the neurologist saw me for the second time on day nine, he said, 'You should have had that MRI when I first suggested it.'

The next day, I finally got an MRI, confirming that I had, in fact, developed acute compartment syndrome. *Finally,* I thought. They had finally concluded that it was compartment syndrome.

When the orthopaedic surgeons came in to see me on day ten, they came with a whole team to my room. By that stage, I felt like some kind of circus act or museum exhibition with the number of doctors coming in and out and checking my leg. The very first thing the orthopaedic specialist said was, 'Sharon, this is the first time I have heard of what has happened to you, and I came immediately when I heard.'

After having a look at my case file and MRI scans and making calls to eminent trauma surgeons around the country, the orthopaedic team decided against doing a fasciotomy. The damage to my muscles and nerves had already been done, and it was too late to prevent any further damage. Opening up my leg at this stage would only increase my risk of infection.

Over the course of my hospital stay, I had become more and more depressed because I wasn't coping. I was in a lot of pain, I was bed-bound, I needed to use bed pans to go to the toilet, and I had this beautiful baby boy in a cot beside me who I couldn't do anything for. I felt useless and hopeless. All I was good for was breastfeeding.

I felt like a failure of a mother. I felt like a failure of a midwife.

Whenever I had visitors, I just covered up my leg because it was so huge and pretended I was okay. All I wanted to do every day and every minute was cry and cry and cry, but I kept putting on a brave face because I couldn't let myself be 'that midwife' who's lost the plot and wasn't holding it all together.

I felt so let down by my own people, people I trusted and thought were doing everything they could for me.

The whole ordeal was horrible. It was supposed to be the happiest time of my life, but it wasn't. I had lost my identity. I wasn't allowed to speak up as a midwife with my own knowledge because, if I did, I was afraid I would be mocked, and they would think, *Oh, it's that midwife who thinks she knows everything.* But on the other hand, when the diagnosis was given to me, it was as if they relied on me to use my own midwifery knowledge to sort myself out.

I had fallen through the cracks of the maternity care system, stuck somewhere between the identity of a professional midwife and unwell patient but never fully being either. I was disempowered and afraid, alone and unsupported.

Chapter 2

After fifteen days of confinement in my depressing jail cell, I was finally set free to take my son home. I had walked into that hospital an independent, capable, and happy expectant mother. I was wheeled out of the hospital with a rollator walking frame, a foot-drop splint, and a new baby I couldn't carry or physically care for.

I went in whole. I came out broken. That's what the hospital did to me.

My parents drove us home to our apartment, only to realise within an hour of being home that I couldn't do anything without assistance.

I suddenly felt so overwhelmed and depressed at my loss of independence in the simplest of activities of daily living. I needed to be cared for around the clock, and my husband had to return to work.

Who would look after me?

Who would look after our baby?

My parents suggested that we stay with them for a short time until I regained some strength in my weak right leg. At that stage, we had only planned to stay there for a few weeks, but as time progressed, it became more and more clear that we needed their help for a long time to come.

I felt like a useless invalid, unable to do what I needed to do as a mother.

My independence and dignity gone. Just like that.

In those precious early days, tarnished by my inability to do anything at all for my baby, I couldn't get up and walk around on my own. Nappy changes, baths, burping after feeds. All of it. I was good for nothing aside from breastfeeding. I was useless, but at least I still had the ability to breastfeed my son. It was the one thing that I could do that no-one else could do for him.

My parents prepared a mattress out in the lounge room where my baby and I would spend the waking hours, where I'd eat my meals lovingly cooked for me by my parents.

Without anyone to help me at night because my husband was working night shifts, my baby slept in a cot in my parents' room. Remembering this always comes with a twinge of grief.

I had always planned on having him sleep in my room in a cot next to my bed. I believed in the benefits of co-sleeping, and this is what I had planned to do with my baby. I never ever planned to have my child in a separate room. I had looked forward to those night-time cuddles and dream feeding my son in bed.

When it was time to breastfeed, my mum or dad would bring Jeremy to me in the middle of the night or help me walk to their room. Oh, how I wish I could have stood up myself, carried him out of his cot, and settled him on my own.

I remember once when I swung my legs off the bed to stand up in the middle of the night, feeling devastated, and I immediately crumpled to the ground as my ankle rolled in on itself. My heart sank as I realised how much my life had changed, how much my physical ability had deteriorated at the hands of the hospital system that failed to provide the care it should have.

It grieves me a great deal when I think of what was taken from me, those precious moments I had achingly longed for but missed out on, those night-time cuddles and dream feeds I was supposed to have with my little baby.

Those days are gone for good. It is a permanent loss that can never be retrieved.

My parents. I don't know how I would have survived without them. They were middle-aged at the time and had already survived raising four newborns during their lifetime. They didn't need to go through this again—the sleepless nights and additional stress of seeing their eldest daughter lose so much at a time when she should have been thriving.

But they never once complained. It was they who so selflessly and lovingly wanted to have my son sleep in their room. They expressly wanted me to get some decent sleep every night so I could heal and recover.

Then there were the never-ending physiotherapy appointments that ate up enormous chunks of my precious time. My rehab treatment was intensive. The consequences of the permanent damage—foot drop, a severely weak ankle, and major balance issues—needed regular and close attention if I was to rebuild any strength in my leg and foot.

With the frequency of physiotherapy and specialist appointments, it became an arduous task to always take my baby with me. I then began the time-consuming task of expressing my breast milk to keep for my baby while my dad took me to all my medical appointments.

Although I needed to change physiotherapists quite a few times—because no-one really knew how to deal with my situation—I slowly regained some strength and control over my ankle, but my independence was still a distant memory.

I was slowly drowning in a tumultuous sea of depressing emotions, ill-equipped to save myself. The capable, independent, and determined woman I once was had faded away … I had lost control of every facet of my life.

From wife and mother, I had been violently thrust into being a dependent child, back under my parents' roof, depending on everyone else for all of my daily needs. *That* was inexplicably difficult to grasp.

I couldn't move around much, so I also gained a lot of weight quickly and spiralled into a deep postnatal depression that I refused to acknowledge and kept hidden to myself. I struggled alone, in silence.

I was a broken mess inside, too afraid to let anyone see the truth: I wasn't coping.

I was angry. Angry at what was happening to me. Angry every day at myself for not being able to care for my son like I wanted to. Angry at the world. Angry at God! *It wasn't meant to be like this.*

What had they done to me? What had they taken away from me? After only a few weeks of coming home, I had yet to feel the full effect of the consequences of untreated ACS on my life. It was only the beginning of the battles I was yet to endure.

One of the many doctors who had been involved in my care attended my first follow-up appointment at the hospital. She sat with me for what felt like an hour and slowly reviewed my medical records with me. Much to my surprise, she encouraged me to look into my medical records further and admitted that this should never have happened.

She couldn't understand why no-one took the initiative to do a fasciotomy when the neurologist initially suspected an acute compartment syndrome. Being only a junior doctor, she didn't have the power to make those decisions, but she strongly suggested that I do everything I could to get a copy of my own medical records and make a complaint to the hospital.

Before this meeting, I had already been suspicious about the care I had received—or lack thereof. This doctor's stance gave rise to many more questions in my mind.

Why was she suggesting this? What was she trying to tell me without actually telling me?

During that time, I shared a lot about my progress on Facebook. As many of my friends and family wanted to know how I was getting along, this seemed the easiest and most time-efficient way to keep everyone updated. I remember one of my friends, who happened to be an obstetrician, commented on one of my updates that she thought I should get a copy of my medical records before they 'mysteriously disappeared'. By this time, more than a few of my friends had already suggested that.

I looked into litigation options against the hospital because of the damage that I had sustained. Never in my career had I thought that I would ever entertain the idea of taking legal action against the healthcare system I was a part of. I battled with this. To sue anyone seemed like a foreign concept that I was uncomfortable with. However, my life had been uprooted and shaken to the very core. I was furious at what had become of my life, bitterly betrayed by the healthcare system I had placed all of my faith in. I had been one of them. I was one of their own, but they had utterly let me down. Ironically, when I was in hospital and friends and family had alluded to the possibility of a lack of proper care, I vehemently defended my carers, telling everyone that I was 'one of their own' and 'I'm getting the best care'.

Having that veil of illusion ripped away so suddenly was almost as painful as losing my independence.

I no longer felt any loyalty to the system that used me, chewed me up, and unceremoniously spat me out. They took away my independence. They robbed me of the early years of motherhood I had so desperately longed for and dreamed of.

I had a fire in my belly.

I called the medical records department and requested a copy of my medical records. I wanted to inspect every entry myself. I knew what had happened to me from my own perspective as the unwell patient on that hospital bed. But I wanted to read from a perspective that saw me as a bed number on a handover sheet. What had they written about me? How did my care go so horribly wrong that it robbed me of my physical ability to attend to the needs and cares of my new baby?

This simple act of getting my records was the beginning of my fight.

My fight for justice.

I had sounded my battle cry.

I had declared war.

Chapter 3

I received a copy of my records fairly promptly and started studying my notes.

Reading through my records left me horrified at the lack of communication between the medical teams that were looking after me. I had been under the care of eight different medical teams: Obstetrics, Anaesthetics, Neurology, Orthopaedic, Surgical, Infectious Diseases *(because they were convinced I had cellulitis!)*, and the Vascular and Trauma teams (through telephone consultation between my doctors and the doctors at the tertiary referral hospital in the district). I was amused to see so many different teams. Amused, but with anger and frustration slowly building.

Each entry I read through left me more furious than the one before. I couldn't get over how poor the care was. It was all over the place, and no-one seemed to know what to do or take control of the situation.

Each entry by a new team/doctor just repeated the previous entry, and it was obvious that no-one was trying to get to the bottom of it. To say I was angry at what I was reading was an understatement. I was enraged. How could they have treated me so poorly when I was one of them? I felt let down, betrayed, and utterly devastated.

In January 2012, I called the hospital to raise my concerns with the patient representative department. My call was transferred to a woman called Elizabeth, and I introduced myself.

'Hi, Sharon! You're the lady who had compartment syndrome in the maternity ward! I know about you.'

There had obviously been talk amongst the hospital about me! I responded, 'Yes, I am, and I am not happy about the care I received.'

I vented my anger and frustration at how I had been treated while in the care of a hospital I trusted. I talked to Elizabeth about my issues with the care I received: I was not listened to, my concerns were dismissed, and my pain had not been taken seriously by many of the people who had looked after me.

Elizabeth was a godsend. She listened. She understood. She knew what I wanted and needed, even before I had figured that out for myself. After all, it was her job to manage the complaints received by that hospital, but the thing that made Elizabeth different was her empathy and people skills. She cared. She really, truly, genuinely cared about the 'person' in the patient. I wasn't a clinical case or a bed number to her. I was a real person who had feelings and expectations of care that had not been met.

Elizabeth asked me to write an email with questions that I wanted answered by the doctors, and if their response wasn't to my satisfaction, she would arrange a meeting between me and the director of medical services.

I got to work and began writing my complaint letter; however, before I had a chance to finish the letter, and much to my surprise, I received a call from Ben Brander, one of the senior managers of the hospital. My insider knowledge of the hospital system told me this was not normal practice. This particular manager wouldn't be calling complainants unless there was something serious happening.

'I am so sorry for what happened to you during your hospital admission,' he began. I didn't know what to say, so I just listened. The call consisted of him telling me that *'it never should have happened'* and he was calling me to let me know he had already submitted an insurance claim. Mr Brander asked me to send all my medical receipts through so they could reimburse me.

That's strange, I thought. I didn't know what was going on and couldn't understand why they already wanted to reimburse me when I was yet to submit my formal written complaint. I discussed my thoughts with Lily, a friend who also happened to be a lawyer. Her perspective was that if the insurance company had already approved my medical claims, they were definitely hiding something from me.

After a lot of thought, consideration, and discussion with family and some close friends, I engaged a lawyer. I didn't have money to pay them upfront, so the only option I had was to use one of those 'only pay if you win' lawyers. With Lily's help, I made a few calls and settled on a small law firm. I was allocated a female lawyer who seemed kind but was somewhat detached and very busy. I had to remind myself that I wasn't hiring her to be a therapist, so it was fine for her to be detached. The main thing was that she knew exactly what ACS was, listened to my story, and commenced a case. To minimise cost, Lily and I put together our own chronology based on the medical records.

Pouring over each written entry of my records exacerbated my anger. I was boiling with rage. Every fibre of my being was at a constant level of fury; every thought was anger. And this anger and frustration was my driving force, fuelling my energy to get some justice. I wanted justice.

I needed justice.

I needed to be heard and acknowledged.

And I needed to fix the system.

Elizabeth knew I wasn't happy with the phone call I had received from Mr Brander, so she had arranged for me to meet with him to discuss my concerns further.

In May 2012, my parents drove me, along with my son, to the hospital, and they came to the meeting to support me. They each sat on either side of me as if to guard me against any further damage and assault to my already fragile mental state. Elizabeth, my advocate, was also there, along with Agnes Ding, a representative from the hospital's Women's and Children's Department.

Agnes opened the discussion by apologising for what had happened to me. 'I'm deeply sorry and would like to apologise on behalf of some of the staff members for not following proper procedures.'

So far, so good, I thought.

Agnes continued, 'I know you've suffered many complications since this happened,' referring to the acute compartment syndrome. 'It is a rare, incredibly rare situation,' she said, and, 'It's a shame you had this complication.'

Ben Brander piped up next. 'I want to echo the same,' he said in what seemed like feigned sincerity, 'and I also want to acknowledge the apology extended to Sharon by me, over the phone.'

I rolled my eyes. *A desperate attempt to draw attention to his gallantry,* I thought. Nevertheless, he deserved to have his say, too.

In a tone screaming of authority, Ben Brander defensively outlined the changes that had been implemented as a result of my 'case'. 'We have conducted an investigation and have now implemented strategies to educate staff and improve practice. We don't really know how this happened, and we may not ever find out how.'

Oh, Lord, can I just get up and leave now? I thought. He hadn't read my complaint letter properly. He had not understood why I was so angry. I wasn't there to find out *how* I developed ACS. I was there to discuss the poor care that led to me not getting the correct emergency treatment for the ACS.

Agnes, interrupting my thoughts, said, 'Unfortunately, acute compartment syndrome is one of the many things on the fine print list for complications in pregnancy, and yours was probably a complication of the pregnancy.'

I opened my mouth, but before I could speak, Agnes' voice sounded again. 'But despite this, you had the very best doctors treating you, and it's just so unfortunate that this happened to you,' she said, seemingly dismissing my accusations of poor medical care.

Everyone in the room looked at me for my reply. I felt both my parents' firm hands resting supportively on my shoulders, reminding me to be brave, reminding me I am not alone.

It was my turn to speak now. I took a deep breath, mustering every fibre of strength to hold back my tears.

Directing my comments to Ben and Agnes, I said, 'I was healthy throughout my pregnancy, driving right up until the last day on my own. I only stopped work early because I had threatened premature labour. The day after I had the baby, I was in agonising pain. No-one was listening to me. The pain was worse than labour, and at that moment, I just wanted to cut my leg off.'

I looked up. Agnes was studying my face carefully. Ben shifted in his chair uncomfortably.

I continued. 'When I lowered my leg, I could feel the blood rushing down. There was so much pressure in my leg that it felt like it was about to burst open. If someone had just listened to me, listened to the magnitude of pain I was in, I can't help but think this wouldn't have happened to me. Not the ACS, but the consequences of the delayed diagnosis. I would have had the emergency fasciotomy and quite possibly wouldn't have sustained the permanent damage to my nerves and muscles.'

Both Agnes and Ben nodded and again apologised for what happened to me, only to redirect the conversation back to their efforts to implement changes.

'I just want to reiterate,' said Ben, 'that we *have* put strategies in place to better care for patients in situations like this.'

'We are educating all staff to think outside the box, outside the sphere of obstetrics, and listen to the patients,' chimed Agnes. 'Again, I want to highlight that this is a rare case, and no-one had ever seen something like this before in the obstetric ward.

'It definitely could have been better managed,' she repeated, 'but if the doctors *were* going to identify the compartment syndrome, they *wouldn't* have needed a pressure test or MRI—they would have gone straight to surgery.'

'Then why didn't they follow up on the neurologist's query diagnosis of acute compartment syndrome that he raised at the very beginning?' I retorted. It was clearly obvious to all in the room that my anger was rising. 'Look,' I said, glaring at Ben and Agnes. 'I am *aware* that people make mistakes, but in *this* situation, *my* situation, someone had already queried what I had. Why wasn't anything done about that query? I mean, it wasn't a junior doctor who had suggested ACS; it was the visiting medical officer, for goodness' sake!' I blurted out, exasperated at them both. 'Why wasn't an MRI done then and there? Why didn't they do a pressure test of the compartments in my leg to rule out compartment syndrome? Was it *that* difficult?'

Agnes and Ben seemed to be at a loss to answer my very specific questions. Frustrated, I asked, 'Which medical team was I under? Who was responsible for my care? There were many teams involved, and by the looks of my medical records, no-one seemed to be taking charge, and no-one was communicating with each other. When the neurologist suggested ACS, who was responsible for organising the tests to investigate that query diagnosis? Who was responsible?'

'You were under the obstetric team,' replied Agnes, 'and you were definitely given the best possible care when this happened.'

'If I was *really* given the best care,' I retorted, 'then why did the surgical team keep treating me for cellulitis when my body *wasn't* responding to the antibiotics? They changed my antibiotics *four* times! Four times! Wouldn't you expect raging cellulitis to respond to the strong antibiotics I was given?'

I continued my exasperated tirade, not giving anyone a second to get a word in. 'Why wasn't the orthopaedic team called in to eliminate compartment syndrome for the query diagnoses made by the neurologist early on? If the orthopaedic team was called in to see me, it might have been possible to save my nerve and muscle.'

Ben Brander, looking even more uncomfortable with my line of questioning, remained silent, so Agnes responded, seeming to carefully consider her words. 'Because you had cellulitis and did not have a fracture in your leg, the vascular team was called, as they were the appropriate team. The orthopaedic team would only have been called in if you had a fracture or some kind of trauma. The neurologist probably didn't *really* think it was compartment syndrome because, if he seriously thought it might be, he would have followed it up himself and ordered the appropriate tests.'

Bull crap, I thought. It wasn't the neurologist's job to follow up on that. He was a visiting medical officer who had been called in for his opinion. He made a few suggestions and would have expected my treating medical team to follow up on the suggested diagnoses.

I was getting nowhere with this dynamic duo.

Agnes continued with her excuses. 'And anyway, by the time the neurologist queried compartment syndrome, it would have already been too late to do a fasciotomy because it should have been done within four hours. That's the crucial time to do a fasciotomy.'

At this point, Ben Brander piped up, 'Again, we think it would have been too late to do anything. I've been talking to your orthopaedic specialist and others about compartment syndrome, and they all said it is very rare for anyone to have this kind of complication after giving birth.'

Again, I rolled my eyes. I wasn't there to question or discuss the rarity of compartment syndrome after giving birth. I was there to address the poor care and their failure to listen to me and take my complaints of pain seriously. That is where they stuffed up. And these two pineapple heads didn't seem capable of understanding. They weren't listening, either.

Frustration levels rising and with tears threatening to flow, I said, 'I'm not happy that I had been treated with some of the strongest antibiotics all that time, only to find out later that I never had cellulitis.'

'Who told you you had compartment syndrome?' replied Agnes, quickly.

'The orthopaedic doctor I saw on my first visit to the clinic after I was discharged from hospital. He said that I never had cellulitis, and if it really *was* cellulitis, then the antibiotics would have definitely treated it.' I had been given ultra-strong IV antibiotics for the fifteen days I was in hospital and discharged home with another two-week course of oral antibiotics. By the time I had gone home, the redness in my leg was still visible. I said, 'The orthopaedic doctor said the redness was from the inflammation caused by the compartment syndrome. *Not* cellulitis. He told me there was no point in continuing to take antibiotics because it wasn't an infection. If it had truly been an infection, then it would have cleared with the amount of strong antibiotics I had been on.'

At this, Agnes and Ben began a debate over what I had actually been diagnosed with.

'The orthopaedic registrar,' said Agnes, 'was wrong to say you didn't have cellulitis. You had all the signs of cellulitis.'

Just a few minutes ago, they were admitting that I had developed a compartment syndrome and, although rare, it should have been better managed. Now I *didn't* have compartment syndrome?

Angrily, I asked, 'When was the diagnosis of cellulitis actually made? Because all throughout my notes, "query cellulitis" is written, and a definite diagnosis was never made. Why wasn't a test done to confirm cellulitis, like a blood culture? How do you make a definite diagnosis of cellulitis? And what about my temperature? If I had an infection such as cellulitis, shouldn't I have had a high temperature? I was afebrile the whole time. Why wasn't anyone suspicious about this?'

'Because you don't need to have a temperature to have cellulitis,' responded Agnes. 'You had all the symptoms of cellulitis, so you definitely had cellulitis. Cellulitis is a bedside clinical diagnosis made by the clinician. There is no test to diagnostically confirm cellulitis.'

I was incensed. *'Then how could the doctors be sure I had cellulitis?'* I blurted exasperatedly. I might have been angry, but I was still able to think clinically.

'Responding to the antibiotics would have confirmed that you had cellulitis,' claimed Agnes, defensively.

What a duo of stupid people, I thought. They didn't know my clinical details properly. It was clear they hadn't read my medical records, because my antibiotics had been changed four times and I hadn't responded to any of them. Knowing I had just caught them out, I calmly replied, 'Just to be clear, as you can see from my medical records, my symptoms did *not* improve with the antibiotics. I still had the redness over the shin area on my right lower leg, and it was still warm to touch after the two-week course of oral antibiotics I had following discharge from hospital. So I had a total of four weeks of strong antibiotics, and my symptoms didn't improve.' I paused for effect. 'So how was that cellulitis?' I asked. I didn't expect a clever answer because it was clear to me that these two had no idea what they were saying.

Resigned to defeat, Agnes replied, 'We will probably never know if you had cellulitis or not.' She sighed.

Somewhere along the way, the tears had broken free and were streaming down my face. I couldn't speak anymore. I was sad, exhausted, and deflated.

Then I heard my mum's bold voice, loud and clear, directed at Agnes and Ben. 'So how can you be sure Sharon didn't have compartment syndrome if you can't say for sure that she had cellulitis? Why could you not have done an MRI to confirm or eliminate it? Why was the orthopaedic team not called to eliminate the diagnosis?'

'Because Sharon didn't have the classic symptoms of compartment syndrome,' replied Agnes. 'Her leg was red, and that is more a symptom of cellulitis, not a symptom of compartment syndrome.'

Oh my goodness! Clearly, she didn't know much about compartment syndrome.

Adamant in her conviction that it *was* cellulitis, Agnes added, 'It may well have been the cellulitis that caused the compartment syndrome. The symptoms of cellulitis and compartment syndrome are similar.'

Gosh, such conflicting information from these two! I thought. *Make up your minds.*

'Then what about the pain I had?' I challenged Agnes. 'Is the level of pain I experienced acceptable for a diagnosis of cellulitis? They gave me morphine, but it didn't touch the pain. Even after fifty-five minutes, when I told the midwives that the morphine hadn't worked yet, the doctors wanted me to wait another twenty minutes for the morphine to take effect. Is that *normal,* Agnes?'

They wanted to be difficult? *Well, two can play at that game,* I thought. I had enough knowledge about medications to know how long it should have taken for the morphine to take effect if it was going to relieve my pain.

'Shouldn't the morphine have worked within twenty minutes and not fifty-five?' I interrogated, staring directly at Agnes. 'Does morphine *really* take that long to work for pain relief?'

Agnes was speechless, so I firmly stated, with conviction, 'The dose of morphine I was given *should* have taken effect within twenty minutes if my body was going to respond to morphine. Clearly, the morphine did not work to relieve the agonising pain I was in.'

'Yes, you're right, Sharon. It should have worked within twenty minutes.' Agnes sighed, seemingly resigned to admitting that I was right. 'Your pain should have been better managed.'

Finally, I thought. *At least she admitted to that!*

Then Ben Brander decided he would contribute to the debate. 'Cellulitis *can* be that painful,' he said, with an air of superiority about him.

'Oh, really?' I asked. 'A pain *that* extreme that I wanted to cut my own leg off? A pain so excruciating that morphine didn't touch it?'

You think you know what compartment syndrome is, do you? I thought to myself. *Then let me hit your leg with a baseball bat hard enough to give you an ACS so you can see for yourself just how painful it is. Then you can come back and tell me that cellulitis is as painful as compartment syndrome.* I wanted to express exactly what I was feeling, but I was enraged. Furious. Too furious to say anything. My emotions got the better of me, and I began sobbing.

After taking a few minutes to compose myself, I spoke again. 'I managed labour so well with minimal pain relief, without requesting an epidural. I only had an epidural because it was suggested to me by my midwife at the very end in order to give me a couple of hours of rest so I would have the energy to push. I managed a posterior labour, which is known to be a very painful labour because of the malposition of the baby's head. Even after the caesarean, a major abdominal surgery, when I got up and out of bed the next morning, I was only having paracetamol and diclofenac. So when I started complaining of extreme pain in my leg, I wasn't joking. Clearly, I have a high pain threshold, and the doctors should have thought of that and taken me seriously, especially considering I had done so well managing my pain in labour.

'Instead, I was not taken seriously. I know their attitudes, as well as some of the midwives who were looking after me, and they didn't believe I was really in that much pain. They dismissed my pain levels. They failed to take me seriously. If their attitudes were different and someone actually listened to me and took me seriously, maybe they could have prevented all the complications that I am dealing with right now. Maybe someone might have organised a further medical review, or maybe someone might have been able to diagnose compartment syndrome sooner and do a fasciotomy.' I knew I had said some of these things before, but I felt Ben and Agnes hadn't really listened to what I had said. I needed to spell it out again for them to understand my point of view. This was not about developing compartment syndrome. I was there, having this meeting, because I had received terribly shocking postnatal care.

After that impassioned speech, I thought I'd finally gotten through to them.

'Diagnoses can sometimes take days to make,' replied Agnes, 'and by the time we made that diagnosis, it would have been too late.'

'And if anyone suspected compartment syndrome,' interjected Ben Brander, 'they wouldn't have even bothered with a pressure test or MRI. They would have immediately done a fasciotomy. It is such a rare condition; I doubt anyone would have picked up on it.'

'Well, I've heard of two cases of non-traumatic compartment syndrome since it happened to me,' I argued. 'One was a patient in a nearby hospital who was diagnosed by a friend's husband, a junior doctor, and the orthopaedic team was called in immediately. Another was a patient who was looked after by my husband, who is a nurse. Both were treated appropriately. So, if *I've* heard of two cases so soon after my case, then it can't be that rare, can it?'

'No, it's not,' admitted Ben Brander, who was obviously caught off guard by my persistence in challenging everything he said.

I then heard my dad's calm voice say, 'While Sharon was in hospital, I saw our GP and described her symptoms to him. At the very first instance, my GP said that my daughter's symptoms sounded like it *was* compartment syndrome.'

Feeling stronger after hearing my dad's voice, I continued on the offensive. 'What would have happened if I had lost my leg, or my life, because of a late diagnosis of compartment syndrome? I am extremely fortunate to have my leg and be able to walk, but a loss of a limb is almost always a consequence of an undiagnosed acute compartment syndrome.' I paused to take a breath. 'What would have happened if I developed renal failure because of the breakdown of muscle in my leg and then needed dialysis? Why wasn't that looked into when I had elevated liver function tests and an elevated creatinine kinase level? Shouldn't that have indicated something to the doctors because my blood results were unusually all over the place?'

'These are all "what if" questions,' said Ben Brander, 'and you *do* still have a leg. Your orthopaedic doctor told me he is very happy with your progress—much better than he initially expected.'

'Firstly,' I replied, 'I didn't give you consent to make calls to find out about my confidential medical progress. And secondly, what would have happened if I *did* lose my leg?' I wanted him to face the reality of the potential outcome I could have experienced. 'It was such a close near miss, and the outcomes would have been drastic if I had lost my leg.'

'Then we would deal with that in a different way,' Ben replied as if to dismiss my point.

'But I'm concerned that this might happen to someone else,' I quickly replied. 'Considering the lack of knowledge the doctors who looked after me seemed to have when it comes to an emergency limb- and life-threatening condition, what if this happens again and another woman loses her leg? Because apparently, diagnoses can take days to make, according to Agnes here.' I turned my head back to Agnes. But I wasn't finished. 'It shouldn't happen like that. My pain should have been addressed, and the doctors treating me should have taken my complaints of pain seriously and treated me immediately! They should know what is and isn't a normal level of pain in women who have had caesareans.'

I still had more to say. 'My orthopaedic specialist said that the pain, which was not relieved by *morphine*, and which was disproportional to the caesarean section, should have been the biggest indicator of compartment syndrome. He said that it seems that everyone involved in my care failed to appreciate the seriousness of it and that if he had been called to see me when I was in hospital, he would have gotten up in the middle of the night for it and rushed to see me. My orthopaedic surgeon told me that the surgical team *should* have been able to identify compartment syndrome.'

Insistent on defending the hospital, Ben Brander retorted, 'But he didn't tell *us* that,' as if to imply that I was in some way making this up.

He could keep defending the hospital all he wanted, but I wasn't about to stop my attack. 'If the orthopaedic surgeon *had* been called in earlier, my muscle and nerve could have possibly been saved. I had foot drop on day two, and I was losing the sensation around the big toe on day four. Why was that not picked up, too? I told the midwife looking after me on day four about the loss of sensation. It's even documented in my medical records, but nothing was done about that.'

'Yes, that should also have been better managed,' replied Agnes.

I didn't stop. I needed to talk and tell them everything. 'Even on day five, when I said how much pain I was in, and when I told them that it was worse than labour, no-one seemed to really listen to me. I know some of the midwives commented and complained about me in handover to other midwives about the amount of times that I was calling the buzzer about my pain, but this was dismissed. One midwife even decided all on her own to change the quantity of pain relief I was given despite the ordered amount of oxycodone—I was not given the proper dosage of oxycodone. I had to look at my medication chart for myself and demand the ordered dosage of oxycodone for the terrible pain I was in. Another midwife had a rude attitude and passed remarks suggesting I would become addicted, and at a later stage, when she heard my baby cry for more than one minute, said that my baby was probably showing signs of withdrawal from "all the high doses of pain medication" I had. I have worked in two tertiary referral hospitals and looked after several babies who were withdrawing. *My* baby was *not* withdrawing.'

At this, Agnes looked genuinely shocked and disappointed to hear that I had been treated like this by some of the staff. 'I am so sorry on behalf of these staff members, and I want to reiterate to you that we are training and educating the staff to better talk to patients and listen to them.'

The conversation then turned to how I felt they failed in their duty of care to ensure I had the appropriate follow-up to manage the outcome. 'I read in the medical records,' I said, 'that I was supposed to have a follow-up with a neurologist when I was discharged, but this had not been done. I wasn't even aware, until I read the records myself, that the neurologist wanted to see me in his private consulting rooms to follow up the nerve issues.'

Ben was quick to exempt the hospital from any responsibility and said, 'This was because the orthopaedic specialist took charge of you.'

Agnes added, 'We can't say anything about that.'

'Okay,' I replied. 'I understand you don't want to take any responsibility for that, but I was just so shocked to discover how poor the communication was between all the care providers I had. *I* was the one who requested my orthopaedic specialist do a nerve conduction study because, while I was in hospital, the neurologist had mentioned it to me and said that if my big toe hadn't improved in ten days, I would need a nerve conduction study. No-one followed up on this in the hospital. I had to initiate all of this myself. It was as if no-one wanted to have any responsibility for ensuring I had a medical care plan following discharge. I had no idea how to manage this myself. The fragmented medical care I received resulted in me falling through the cracks of this healthcare system.

'My biggest disappointment,' I said, 'was that no-one was listening to me.'

I then began to explain the way I was delivered the diagnosis of compartment syndrome at two o'clock in the morning and how I was expected to rely on my own clinical knowledge while I was in so much pain. 'She didn't have any clue about compartment syndrome, and the only answer she had for me was "I don't know". When she told me that the MRI confirmed acute compartment syndrome and that the surgeons would only come to see me the *next* morning, and knowing that ACS should be dealt with immediately, I was devastated. I was terrified I would lose my leg before the surgeons could come to see me. My mum had to call my husband and my dad in the middle of the night because I was such a mess and so upset. Is *this* the acceptable way to inform a patient of such a frightening diagnosis?'

I could tell that my words were affecting Agnes. She had appeared to soften in her manner toward me and kindly replied, 'I am sorry for the way you were given your diagnosis. I wasn't aware that this was an issue for you, but this is definitely not the right way to communicate a diagnosis like compartment syndrome to a patient, especially one with a medical understanding of the urgency of it. And it definitely should not have happened at that time of night.'

After taking some time to think, Agnes made a reflective statement. 'Could we have prevented it? No. Obstetricians have never seen compartment syndrome in this context.'

By this point, I was completely and utterly drained.

In a calm and composed nature characteristic of my dad, he slowly said, 'It is all good for you to apologise and wash your hands of it all, but what about my daughter? What are you all going to do to help her?'

I was thankful for my dad's wisdom and good sense in asking this question.

My dad continued, 'My daughter is a young woman who cannot go back to the normal job that she is trained for in this condition. What is her future? What are you going to do to help her?'

Ben Brander, suddenly sounding confident again, replied by asking, 'What would you like us to do?'

'You need to support her,' said my dad. 'She will need surgery in the future, and who is going to pay for that? We are not asking for millions of dollars here, but she needs to be compensated and supported financially in all her medical expenses.'

'As I said before on the phone to Sharon,' replied Ben, 'the offer still stands to pay out-of-pocket medical costs. As soon as Sharon contacted the hospital, I immediately sent over your case to the hospital insurance, and they are going to pay out-of-pocket expenses.' As if this would solve all my problems, he said, 'Keep the receipts, and we will reimburse you, but we don't have an unlimited slush fund, so even this needs to be quantified. It can't be an ongoing cost. We only have money in the scope of a few thousand, and definitely not in the tens of thousands. We can pay some, but it is limited to the amount we can offer.'

'What about the surgery I will need?' I asked. 'I want to have the very best surgeon because I need to have the best possible outcome for my future, and I know it will not be cheap.'

Ben repeated, 'We have a limited amount we can give.'

Feeling dejected and exhausted, I had nothing more to say.

'Two things need to happen here,' my mum said. 'One—Sharon needs to be compensated for what happened to her. She has gone through a lot, and she needs help with the surgery costs and recovery. The other is that medical practices need to be improved so this won't happen to anyone else, especially a young woman like Sharon.'

'Unfortunately,' Ben replied, 'we don't have money—a slush fund or a compensation system—in this state, so what we can do is limited and needs to be quantified.'

'I understand you are saying that from the management point of view,' my mum replied. 'We know you have boundaries to work within, and we can also understand what you are saying and why you are saying these things. But you need to understand that Sharon needs to do what is best for her, and we hope you appreciate and understand that.' My clever and intuitive mum was referring to litigation, giving them a heads up we were going to come for them.

Both Ben Brander and Agnes Ding indicated that they understood what my mum had warned them of, and both of them apologised again for what had to experience.

'Clearly, this whole ordeal has greatly affected you, Sharon,' I heard Agnes say. 'I suggest getting some counselling to help you work through all of this.'

Who's going to pay the exorbitant cost for the counselling I would need to get over all of this? I thought. She can make all the suggestions she wants, but she gets to go back to her life at home, and I will become a distant memory for her. A clinical case. Nothing more. Yet I will have to keep living with the consequences, and I don't get to just forget it all. As I left the room, I overhead Elizabeth say, '*Is* she going to receive any compensation for all of this? She's been through hell and is still going through hell.'

'It would be years before she actually gets anything back,' I heard Ben say.

I was starting to realise the hopelessness of my situation.

Chapter 4

The meeting with Ben Brander and Agnes Ding catapulted me into a spiral of panic about my future career. I enjoyed catching babies, but most of all, I loved looking after women and babies in the postnatal wards. I loved the satisfaction and joy I got when I helped a new mum successfully breastfeed her baby. I loved teaching new mums and dads how to bathe, swaddle, and settle their new baby. I remember the joy of teaching new fathers how to change their baby's nappy and watching them 'get it' when they did it for the first time. It was such a special time, and I always felt so privileged and honoured to be a part of these moments.

Deep in the trenches of my gut, however, I knew that my clinical career in midwifery and nursing was over. Working as a clinical midwife meant being able to stand on my feet for long periods of time, run to an emergency, and keep my balance while holding other people's precious babies. I could barely stay on my feet longer than fifteen minutes at a time, and I was frequently losing my balance and falling.

It was a risk that I was not willing to take, and I was sure no employer would be willing to take it either. Facing the very real prospect of never being able to catch babies and work as a clinical midwife again, the profoundness of my loss dawned on me. I mourned the loss of my career plans, but I was determined to turn my situation into something positive.

But how could I do this? I had nothing else under my belt. No other qualifications. All I knew was nursing or midwifery. I didn't have any admin or office experience. Nothing. Unlike many of my friends, I hadn't even worked at McDonald's as a teenager.

Nevertheless, something stirred inside me. I had determination and too much of a fighting spirit to let this kick me to the ground.

I had dreamed of one day working for the World Health Organization. My passion for global maternal health had seen me enrol in a Master of Public Health (MPH) and Master of International Public Health (MIPH) during the second half of 2011, while I was still pregnant.

I knew what I had to do, so I threw myself into completing my studies. Having only finished two subjects at that stage, I quickly enrolled in distance learning and resolved to work hard to put myself in a position where I could get a non-clinical job.

Those days were hard. I was studying for two master's degrees, dealing with the hospital, and having regular medical and physiotherapy appointments, all while learning to be a mum and on top of navigating a marriage that was slowly deteriorating from the weight of trauma thrown on it.

I was having nightmares and flashbacks to having a swollen, painful leg, but at the same time, I was in complete denial about these symptoms of post-traumatic stress disorder (PTSD). While I knew I wasn't okay, I simply didn't have time for PTSD! My plate was overflowing with university assignments, motherhood, and rehab. There were many sleepless nights, but I pushed myself. I needed this. Once my son would sleep, I'd get my computer out and work. Before I knew it, it was time for another breastfeed. Then I would be back to working on my assignments.

I was determined to make something of myself and not let what happened to me be the end of me. I was exhausted, but I kept pushing through my master's degrees.

I was also acutely aware that I needed some kind of work experience that was not clinical nursing or midwifery. At the time, I was still permanently employed (by the hospital I worked at before I took maternity leave), but I was really worried that I would be forced to resign from my position once my maternity leave was finished. The only solution was to find a volunteering position somewhere. I didn't care where; I just needed something I could learn and broaden my experience with.

I did some googling and came across the World Health Organization Collaborating Centre (WHOCC) for nursing and midwifery, and, to my surprise, it was located at the

University of Technology Sydney building! Perfect. I had completed my Bachelor of Nursing at the city campus there. I contacted them, and the director asked me to come in to meet her. That week, I made my trek into the city to meet the director. We had a pleasant chat, and I started there straight away.

My son was only five months old at the time, and my leg was not very strong, but I felt I could manage two trips into the city each week, so I offered to volunteer twice a week. Thankfully, a lot of this work was done from home.

It started off as an unpaid research assistant/intern position, but after the director saw my dedication and commitment to the position, she found some extra funds and started paying me, and I was given the official title of 'Intern'. I was elated by this.

Through volunteering, I was able to gain experience in administrative, research, and other non-clinical skills that I previously did not have. By the end of my time there, the director wrote me a stellar letter of recommendation on the World Health Organization letterhead, detailing all the work I had done for them. I proudly keep this in my CV now.

Not long after staring at the WHOCC, I received a letter from the hospital in response to my initial complaint, which included a summary of the meeting we had in May. I wasn't happy with their stance, and while I knew Elizabeth did her best to resolve my complaints, I wasn't satisfied that Ben Brander and Agnes Ding had listened to me, really listened with empathy and understanding, and acknowledged what their stuff-up had cost me. Their letter was defensive.

I didn't want defensive. I wanted acknowledgement of what this had cost my life. Not financially—I didn't even care about that. But personally, as a mother, wife, daughter, and midwife. The loss of identity is so profound, and I don't believe it can be truly quantified. I wanted them to know what I had lost and to listen and understand what my life had become. Even though, at that time, it had not even been a year since the ACS, the impact was enormous. If I had known then just how much more my life would continue to be impacted, and all the trauma that was yet to come because of this, I don't think I would have survived.

To them, I was just a 'case'. When I was in hospital, I was nothing more than a bed number. A clinical complication. They see me for a few days while I am in hospital. They deal with the unfortunate complications, but then they go home to their own families and come back to work for a new set of clinical patients. The obstetric patient with compartment syndrome becomes a distant memory to them.

But for me, I had to live with the consequences of their medical care, or lack thereof, every day. Life goes on for me, too, but acute compartment syndrome and its long-term complications wasn't a distant memory for me. It was my very real present. And I needed them to know this. I needed to remind them of the importance of listening to their patients because once patients are sent home, they have to keep living with the consequences of their care or lack thereof. In addition to the never-ending physical pain, my life was impacted in many ways.

Sometimes, my parents would take me out to have coffee just to get me out of the house. I used to get stared at a lot in public. I had a little baby, but I was walking around with a walking frame and a foot-drop splint. It was an embarrassment to leave the house like that.

I had to wear the splint at all times, even when I was sleeping, and to keep the splint in place, I had to wear a large sock over it.

I couldn't even wear nice shoes with a pretty dress. This might seem frivolous, but there was a time when it was a real issue for me and impacted my own feelings of being feminine.

But what I wanted the hospital to understand the most was how it significantly affected my experience of motherhood. I needed them to listen to me, to understand how their stuff-up restricted me from doing all the things for my son that I desperately wanted to do and how deeply painful that loss was to me.

Before I had given birth, baby-wearing was something I was obsessed with. My friend Lily had bought me an Ergo sling for my baby shower, and I had been so excited to use it. When I was pregnant, I couldn't wait to use this sling and carry my little one around. It would be a wonderful thing to continue being independent while my child was snuggled at my chest. I was desperate to experience the bonding that baby-wearing would facilitate.

I had dreamed of going for long walks during the day, socialising with new mothers, and doing all the things I needed to do around the house while wearing my baby in the sling.

I never got to even go to the supermarket for grocery shopping with my baby in my sling. I know these activities sound like mundane chores that many others might see as a burden, but I longed to do these things with my baby at my chest.

In the early years of my son's life, when I saw mothers at the shopping centre with their children in a sling or on the seat of the trolley, I felt a twang of grief for the loss of those parts of motherhood that I never got to experience with my son. Even now, ten years later, when I'm out and about with my son and I see a mamma with a baby at her chest, I instinctively wrap my arms around my son and hold him a little closer.

Socially, the physical restriction was a catastrophe for me. I had longed to attend mothers' groups and meet new mums and make friends with others who had babies my son's age. During my pregnancy, I had been really excited about this. None of my friends had babies at the time, so it was an exciting prospect to meet new mums and their bubs. Unfortunately, I never got to join a mothers' group because of the physical restrictions that prevented me from driving and going out with my baby on my own.

It was a rite of passage that I missed out on.

But more than the physical pain and limitations, my inability to care for my son on my own, to just be his mother and attend to all the tasks that a mother should be able to do, caused more internal pain and grief than all the other things.

The thing that really crushes my heart, even to this day, is that when he cried, it was someone else who ran to him to pick him up out of his cot and settle him back to sleep on their chest in their arms, not mine. Even though it was my own family who happily attended to every one of my son's needs, it wasn't *me.* It should have been me. *I* should have been the one to respond to his cries and rock him to sleep in my arms. It was *supposed* to be me. It should have been *my* face that he saw first when he cried. But it wasn't. I couldn't get up fast enough to run to him.

I remember working night shifts on the postnatal wards, putting other women's babies to sleep, rocking them in my arms, pacing corridors with them, longing for a time when it would be my own baby that I was putting back to sleep in my arms, against my chest. But when that time came, it wasn't me who did that for my child. I had to watch others comfort and reassure my baby, and it grieves me that I couldn't do it. This causes so much heartache for me. This is the loss that I *still* have a hard time coming to terms with.

Because I can never get that back.

Many important aspects of motherhood were taken away from me that I can never get back. I feel I was robbed of a very important stage of my life and my son's life, all because of their failure to listen to me when I complained of pain in my leg. That failure to listen to me and believe me and do something about it cost me so much of what was precious to me.

I wanted the hospital to know this. I *needed* them to know this and acknowledge all they took from me when they chose to not listen to me when I was a birthing woman in their hospital. In some way, I wanted them to *feel* the pain I was feeling, to experience the same loss and empathise with me for what I had lost.

After all I had been through, the hospital's response letter simply was not good enough. I wasn't sure what to do next, but I knew I'd think of something to make them listen, to make them understand, and to make them apologise for what their care had cost me.

Chapter 5

Life continued, and by early 2013, I eventually completed my dual master's degrees.

At a global health conference I was attending fairly soon after finishing, I bumped into a former professor of mine. We got to talking, and he ended up offering me some work as a research assistant for a project he was conducting at the university. I gratefully accepted his gracious offer and officially began my career in the world of public health research.

Meanwhile, I continued communicating with the lawyers. They were working on my case, albeit extremely slowly. They had obtained at least one expert opinion in support of my case, and they were waiting on another. They made it clear that faster progress would only come with upfront payment, so I was forced to be patient.

Each interaction with the lawyers left me emotionally drained. Whether it be by phone or in face-to-face meetings in their office, discussing my situation never failed to trigger a continuous fountain of tears for weeks at a time.

The challenge of taking legal action against the hospital was learning to survive the roller coaster of emotions that came with it. One minute I would be elated, feeling like I was getting somewhere with my case, and before the very next breath, I would have the rug pulled out from beneath me, sending me into a downward spiral.

I had turned into an emotional wreck, a shell of the person I once was, trying to hold it all together while the insides of me had shattered into a million little pieces.

I couldn't understand what had happened to me. It didn't help that over the previous twelve months, I had gradually developed Volkmann's contractures in my toes, despite intensive physiotherapy. The dead muscles in my lower-right leg had turned to scar tissue, which caused contractures of my ankle and toes. Unfortunately for me, I had developed a severe case of this unwanted complication of untreated acute compartment syndrome. My toes were curling upwards too much, so my foot wouldn't fit into closed-in shoes.

Tendon-lengthening surgery was the only solution, so in February 2013, my expertly skilled orthopaedic surgeon performed the delicate surgery to lengthen my tendon with sheer precision. He lengthened my contracted toes just enough to wear shoes but kept some of the contracture to keep me from tripping over my toes. This 'toe drop' was one of the many consequences of my crushed peroneal nerve. The peroneal nerve was dead from the knee all the way down to my big toe, so in addition to having major balance issues, I also had no control of that big toe. I needed to have some of the contracture still in place to hold that big toe upwards; otherwise, I'd be a walking disaster!

Although the operation had been a success, surgically, it was the first time I had been in hospital since the compartment syndrome.

In the pre-op anaesthetic bay, when the surgeon came to see me before the operation, I remember asking him, 'Is this going to happen to me again?'

Knowing exactly what I was afraid of, he gently took my hand, gave it a tight squeeze, and said calmingly, 'I promise I won't let it happen to you again.'

It wasn't the compartment syndrome that I was afraid of. I was more afraid of the consequences, being in pain and not being listened to, than the ACS itself. And he knew that. He put my mind at ease, promising to make sure my legs were closely monitored during and after the operation.

'If anything happens, no-one is going to dismiss your pain while I'm around,' he said, and I was grateful for this kind, caring, and empathetic surgeon who made me feel safe.

Although my fears had been pacified before the surgery, I remember the nurses speaking to me as I awoke from the fog of anaesthetic sleep, asking, 'Sharon, do you feel any pain?'

'Where's my leg?' I drowsily replied. 'My leg! Is my leg there?' Right there on that hospital bed, my mind had transported me back to when the ACS started.

I remember hearing someone say, 'She had acute compartment syndrome that wasn't treated, so she's scared of it happening again.'

Shortly after that comment, I remember a calming voice saying, 'It's okay, Sharon. Your legs are both here, and they are fine, and nothing has happened to them. The surgery went well.'

That night in hospital, my leg was thickly wrapped up in a bandage, resting under a bed cradle to keep the weight of the blanket off the operation site. My surgeon had come to see me and reassured me that everything had gone according to plan and that I would be okay, but my mind was racing. I could *feel* my leg blowing up like it had that night in hospital when the ACS started. It *wasn't* blowing up, but it felt so real. Of course, it was all in my head. The bandages around my leg were giving me flashbacks to the night I removed the compression stockings, only to have my leg balloon within seconds.

I was silently freaking out, but I didn't dare press the buzzer to tell the nurses. I was afraid of being treated the same way I had before. I remained silent, a prisoner in my own head. I closed my eyes and prayed to God that my leg wouldn't swell up again.

I ignored those early signs of PTSD. It was just not something I had time, space, or energy to deal with.

When the nurse did come in to check on me later that night, I still didn't share my fears with her and simply asked for pain relief. With silent tears soaking my pillow, eventually, I fell into a codeine-induced sleep.

I woke up the following morning, grateful that I didn't develop compartment syndrome overnight, although there was no reason for it to happen again. What a relief! I was ready to go home, but I needed some kind of walking aid. After trying out a few different types of crutches, I settled on a knee walker. Somewhat like a scooter, this two-wheeled contraption allowed me to rest my operated knee at a ninety-degree angle on a comfortable slab while my left leg scooted along the ground. It was definitely more comfortable than having crutches digging into my armpits.

With my right leg wrapped in a bandage, I was discharged later that morning with strict instructions to remain non-weight-bearing and keep my leg elevated for ten days. On my way home, my parents stopped by a chemist to hire some equipment. I needed a shower chair, a footrest for the shower, and a bed cradle.

Recovery from this operation was difficult. I was pretty much in bed with my leg elevated most of the time, needing full assistance with everything. All over again.

My son, who was only fifteen months at the time, kept coming to me and laying on my chest. I think he knew something was wrong. All I wanted to do was carry him, but I couldn't, so I kept him on my chest or as close to me as possible while I spent my days either in bed or lying on the couch.

Ten painful recovery days later, my surgeon removed the bandage and left the wound uncovered to allow it to heal. By this time, I had muscle wasting again. Ten days of not bearing weight on my right leg were enough to waste away the little muscle I had managed to rebuild over the previous fifteen months. I could do nothing to prevent it, and I knew it was only about to get worse because I had been fitted into a moon boot and had to stay non-weight-bearing for another month.

The following month of recovery wasn't as bad as I had expected, however, as I had gotten used to the knee walker a little more and was able to at least use the bathroom on my own. However, that month set me back a lot in terms of rehab. The weakness in my right leg, along with the associated balance problems, meant I had to learn to walk all over again.

And I had to overcome my fear of driving, which had developed since the ACS.

Chapter 6

Meanwhile, I had remained in regular contact with Elizabeth. I knew Elizabeth was working hard behind the scenes, although I didn't feel I was getting anywhere with my complaint to the hospital.

After I had recovered from the tendon-lengthening surgery, my surgeon cleared me for non-clinical desk work. I got in contact with the manager of the postnatal ward, but they still didn't have anything suitable for me to come back to. My work kept me on extended sick leave, and I was grateful that I could keep my permanent position with them.

Eventually, in August 2013, I came across an expression-of-interest advertisement for a secondment position in the Public Health Unit (PHU) of the same local health district I was employed at. Having recently completed a dual master's in public health, this opportunity was perfect for me to get my foot in the door of the public health world.

The job was normal office hours and desk work! No long shifts on my feet. I applied for the position and got it immediately! I was elated. That week, I started my part-time secondment at the PHU. Although the job paid less than I had been receiving prior to maternity leave, it was still better than nothing! After all, I was starting my career out from scratch again, so I couldn't complain.

I also loved the job.

The secondment was initially meant to be a six-month contract, but it got extended at my request—I *really* loved it.

Eventually, whoever I had been filling in for returned to the office, so the director of nursing transferred me to the Patient Safety and Quality Unit (PSQU). I was to be the acting patient safety and quality manager for Critical Care Services for three days a week. It was a completely new role for me and one that I was unprepared for. I had a lot of learning to do, but I liked new challenges. The pay was much better, but most of all, it was an eye-opener for me.

A real game-changer!

This new role taught me how to deal with patients' complaints and manage incidents that happened in the hospital. I saw the process from the inside.

And I didn't like what I saw.

People wrote complaint letters to the hospital, and my role was to contact the doctors or nurses involved to let them know. The clinicians would then respond in writing and ensure that their staff would receive education and/or further training to prevent a similar incident from occurring again.

Often, the healthcare staff involved would feel deeply sorry for the hurt and pain caused to the patient. I saw genuine, heartfelt apology letters sent back to the PSQU, only to have them shredded to bits by the higher bureaucratic powers and rewritten defensively, erasing all evidence of an actual apology. This didn't happen all the time, but it happened a lot.

I was distraught. Having written a complaint letter to the hospital I gave birth in, I *knew* all these people wanted was to be heard, be acknowledged, and receive a sincere apology.

Angry and frustrated, I was *sure* this was exactly what had been done with my own letters.

This realisation broke me. I felt like I was fighting a losing battle. How could I, little me, fight against the giants of the higher powers of a highly defensive healthcare system? How on earth was I going to get them to listen to me, hear me, acknowledge me, and say sorry to me?

One day, I shared my story with a colleague who worked there.

'Write to the Health Care Complaints Commission,' he said. 'If you go through that avenue and the complaint comes from the HCCC, the hospital would be forced to respond.'

Oh! What a golden nugget of information *that* was! My colleague explained the process and what would happen if I got the HCCC involved. After all, this is exactly what we were doing in the PSQU as well.

I was beside myself with excitement. I could finally see another avenue to get what I wanted. I went home that day with renewed determination and enthusiasm to make the hospital acknowledge all they had done and the impact it had had on my life.

I started writing a new letter. The frustration of not being heard, of not getting the answers I needed, fuelled me to keep going. I started doing my research. I called friends at other maternity units across the local health district to obtain copies of their local policies and protocols. I systematically aligned every moment of my care, every action or lack of, with a corresponding policy they were required to adhere to.

I questioned their care.

I reasoned my points.

I argued my case.

And I supported all of my points with their own policies. I provided all my evidence as to why I was right. I made it clear that I wanted the appropriate processes implemented to prevent this breakdown of care from ever happening again.

Once my letter had been received by the HCCC, the case manager allocated to my complaint informed me that one of their in-house obstetricians had seen ACS following childbirth.

'Has the case been published?' I asked. 'Because I haven't found any other published case reports of it happening in Australia.'

'No, it was never published,' she said.

I began to wonder how many women had actually experienced ACS following childbirth. I had extensively searched for case reports in the medical literature and had come across some published cases, but it was still considered a rare complication. I wondered if it would be more recognised by maternity care staff if every single ACS case was published in the literature. So far, my search of the medical literature had only uncovered cases where obstetricians *had* identified the ACS early and performed an emergency fasciotomy. I found a case published in a legal journal where the obstetrician had not identified the ACS, which had resulted in the woman suffering permanent damage. She had sued the hospital and won a sum of money. Unfortunately, I couldn't find this particular case documented in the medical literature.

Going through the HCCC was also arduous. I could easily have given up. Like dealing with lawyers regarding my case, this also took a very long time. Sometimes, months would pass by before I received an email or telephone call from my case manager regarding the progress of my case investigation.

The lawyers also dealt me a hard blow. One day, they called me into the barrister's chambers to give me an update on my case. I had started off with a very switched-on female lawyer who knew and understood the significance of untreated ACS. After taking on my case, she moved law firms and left me in the hands of an unsympathetic male lawyer who didn't seem to have any sense of urgency to progress my case. 'We're in a good position to win your case,' he said, 'but we are a small firm, and if we are going to take on a local health district, we will need more money and upfront payments to keep going.'

My heart sank. I didn't have the kind of money they were asking for.

He said, 'You are more than welcome to take your case to another firm more capable of taking on a big health organisation head-on, and if you do, we will arrange a transfer of all the paperwork to their office.'

I couldn't believe their audacity. How did they think I would be able to pay them? To add insult to the injury, the lawyer continued, 'But if you win through the other firm, we will still be entitled to take some of your profits for the work we have done here.'

Screw them all! I went home, furious with the lawyer for dragging my case on for so long only to tell me he wanted more money to keep fighting. He also had the nerve to tell me I needed to 'move on'. The lawyer went on to explain that he and his wife had experienced a traumatic birth and, because of that, he understood what I was going through. 'We both considered taking the legal path as well, but it was just best to let it go and move on with life. And that's what I am encouraging you to do, too.'

At that moment, I felt the rage pump through my veins. My blood was boiling. I could have screamed so loud. I wanted to scream until I turned blue. What on earth could *he* possibly understand about what *I* was going through? How dare he tell me to move on? *The patriarchy strikes again,* I thought.

The next day, I made some enquiries and set the wheels in motion to have my case transferred to a different, much bigger, and better-resourced law firm that specialised in medical negligence. I didn't have much money for this endeavour, but I had an official expert opinion from an orthopaedic surgeon in support of my case. I didn't care how long it took; I was determined to take legal action against the hospital. They refused to listen to me when I was a patient. They refused to acknowledge me when I made a complaint. I would *make* them listen to me some way or another, and if litigation was the only way, then so be it. I was adamant to do whatever it took to make them listen, make them understand, and hold them accountable. I was prepared to climb mountains to force a change in the system so that no other woman would have to suffer as I did.

Through all of it, I received unending support and words of praise from friends and extended family for being 'so strong and graceful' and 'always smiling and holding it together'.

But I wasn't holding it together.

None of them knew the truth. No-one knew how broken and shattered I was on the inside. I was in what felt like a permanent state of depression, silently crying in the shower every day when no-one could see me. My heart was dying to get back those moments I missed out on with my baby while at the same time knowing that I never could.

The time I lost with my child, those things I never got to do, never being able to rock my baby back to sleep in my own arms in the middle of the night—I will never get those things back. No amount of money from litigation could ever bring back that time for me to redo.

During those early years, I felt inadequate. In so many ways, I felt like I had failed him as a mother. I was so afraid that our bonding, that important connection between mother and baby, had been affected and severely impaired beyond repair. At the time, my grief and heartache over this loss, so profound and deep, took over my life. It was all I could think about. The knowledge I had about the importance of bonding would often take over my mind, and I would sit in fear of what damage I had done to my son by not being the one who attended to his every need at such a young age.

Ten years on, I know I have an iron-clad bond with my son, but I was left with the feeling that I need to make up for the lost time—for the things I didn't get to do, for the times I didn't get to have him in my room as a baby, for the times I wasn't the one who woke up to the sound of his cry in the middle of the night and rocked him back to sleep in my arms.

Over the years, I have worked through a lot of these issues, but in some way, I still feel a deep sense of loss and a need to make up for what was lost.

Chapter 7

Life continued, as it has to.

After what felt like a lifetime, I finally received a response from the hospital through the HCCC. I read the letter.

Again, I was not impressed.

Many of the points I had raised were left unaddressed. Even clinical details about my birth were incorrect. I couldn't help but feel like the letter was one giant excuse and not an admission or acknowledgement of their failure to provide proper care for me.

I knew then that the things I had seen happen at the PSQU were exactly what happened here.

I was angry and I felt deflated, but I would *not* be defeated. I had fought too hard and come too far to give up now. By this point in time, I was one empowered woman. I had learned about the system through my time at the PSQU. I knew I needed to keep pushing and fighting, not only for myself but for the women who are failed time and time again by our maternity care system. I knew what my mission was. I knew what I had to do. If they were adamant about hiding behind excuses, I decided I was going to take them to court. I even (briefly) entertained the idea of a one-person protest out the front of the hospital to deter anyone from walking into that maternity unit!

My case manager knew I wasn't impressed with the hospital's response and immediately initiated the process for a conciliation meeting.

I couldn't care less about that. *They can arrange a conciliation meeting,* I thought. They could do whatever the hell they wanted.

I was going full steam ahead with litigation.

By the end of 2014, I had secured a permanent position in a PHU as a public health nurse/communicable disease surveillance officer. My marriage was on the verge of breakdown by this time, the consequences of the trauma playing out to destroy so much of what was precious to me.

Somewhere along the way, this disaster got the better of us. I've heard that trauma either makes a relationship or breaks it.

It broke mine.

My marriage ended, and by early 2015, I became a single mother.

Not long after that, I was given a date for my conciliation meeting with the hospital, and my HCCC case manager and I began putting together an agenda for everything we would like to discuss at the meeting. I was sceptical that we would have any success. After all, it had been four long years, and I still hadn't received a proper acknowledgement or a genuine apology from them. There was no evidence to indicate that I would suddenly get one now. But it was my one last shot at talking to the hospital nicely to get what I wanted before I blasted them with litigation.

Elizabeth and I spoke many times over the following months. I was hesitant to attend this meeting, but she eventually managed to convince me it would be a good thing for me to attend.

I spent some time preparing a list of questions to ask them. This was their last chance to get it right, to redeem themselves. I told myself that if this meeting didn't result in me getting what I wanted, I would keep fighting via the lawyers and sue them to hell and back.

When the day of the meeting arrived, my good friend, Lily, came with me to take notes. We parked the car, and I called Elizabeth to let her know I had arrived.

I was surprised by how anxious I was.

When I saw Elizabeth, I burst into tears. I didn't want to go in. I didn't want to talk to them. I was *scared*. What if they dismissed me like they had all this time? What if they played their power games on me? What if they belittled me and my clinical knowledge? These were the thoughts going through my head. They were doctors, and they were there in that meeting to defend their actions. Who was I but an insignificant, upset complainant? *Gosh, what happened to all my courage?* I had no fear while writing those complaint letters, but when it came time to face the people responsible for my pain and trauma, I was terrified.

Elizabeth sat with me and consoled me. She encouraged me to go into the room and promised she would sit next to me and speak if I couldn't.

So, with a tear-streaked face and Lily and Elizabeth, two incredible women, by my side, I mustered the courage to walk into the meeting room.

There were already four people sitting at the large table inside the room.

Elizabeth began by introducing them to me. Dr Michael White was from the Obstetrics and Gynaecology Department, Judy Arrow from Clinical Policy Development, and Dr Richard Smith from the Orthopaedic Department.

The HCCC case manager, Marilyn, who was sitting at the head of the table, commenced the meeting. She welcomed us to the meeting and briefly mentioned what we would discuss before she turned to me and let me start expressing my concerns.

I spoke.

I cried.

I spoke some more.

It was finally my chance to let it all out. I was finally allowed to tell them every detail of how my life had been turned upside down by what happened to me when I was a birthing woman in their maternity unit. The people in the room respectfully remained silent and focused their attention on me while I described in detail my pain, both physical and emotional.

I told them they robbed me of parts of motherhood that I could never get back.

I told them all of it. The loss of my marriage, my career, and my independence.

I don't know how long I spoke but finally, I had let it all out. Finally, I had spoken, and they had been silent, intently listening to every word I said.

Then it was their turn to speak.

Dr White spoke first. 'Sharon, I want to sincerely apologise for what you have gone through. We are all parents, and we couldn't begin to imagine going through what you have gone through.'

It was Ms Arrow's turn to speak, and she also delivered a genuine apology, but I couldn't help but notice Dr Smith's irritability at being there. He appeared impatient and couldn't seem to detach himself from his phone. It couldn't be more obvious that he saw this meeting as a total waste of time. I was tempted to say something about his rudeness, but this wasn't my battle, so I chose to ignore him.

Instead, I focused my attention on Dr White. He spoke so kindly to me. The way he spoke conveyed genuine sorrow for what had happened to me, and this caught me off guard. I'd walked into that room ready for a fight, but he stopped me in my tracks. I wasn't expecting this, but I quickly regained my composure, looked at my notes, and focused my mind on what I was there for.

I directed them to the letter I sent via the HCCC. 'What about all the points I raised in my letter? Why didn't I get a response to all of those points in the hospital's reply? Why wasn't I transferred to the tertiary referral hospital when they realised they weren't equipped to deal with the complication I developed? Why hadn't my doctors followed protocol on so many occasions?'

I was exasperated and exhausted.

After taking a deep breath, Dr White picked up my letter, looked me in the eye, and quietly and softly said, 'You're right, Sharon. Everything you wrote in this letter is right. We stuffed up. We made mistakes. This shouldn't have happened to you.'

The room filled with silence as everyone looked to me for my response.

Suddenly, I could breathe again. Just like that, an enormously heavy weight had lifted off me. With tears streaming down my eyes, I couldn't find my voice.

Dr White continued. He had been on leave at the time I gave birth and said, 'If I had been there, your care would certainly have been managed differently.'

Although I had been angry at everything, listening to Dr White softened me a little. I could tell he meant what he said. I believed him. Finally, I had received the acknowledgement and genuine apology that I had been longing for.

I couldn't believe this had happened. How wonderful it felt to breathe again. It was not until that moment that I became cognizant of the weight of the burden I had been carrying all these years and how much it had been suffocating me. My heart flooded with gratitude for this apology.

This was open disclosure, and finally, the hospital got it right.

'What do you want?' came Dr White's soft voice, interrupting my thoughts.

I hadn't been prepared for the apology, but this question, I had prepared for. I regained my composure and put my professional hat on. I had a whole monologue prepared to convince them to give me what I wanted. I began explaining my point of view to them. 'I'm lucky, but the next woman might not be. The next delayed diagnosis could result in an amputation, as is usually the case for undiagnosed compartment syndrome. All of my doctors thought I wouldn't be able to walk again without a foot-drop splint, and now they can't believe that I can. The neurologist said I had age on my side, but what if the next woman who this happens to doesn't have the same things going for her, like the support I had, the ability to advocate for myself and seek medical care? This happened to me because no-one in obstetrics knew what it was. And no-one could believe it when it was suspected by the neurologist on day two. They couldn't believe it because they hadn't *seen* it in obstetrics. They were not aware of the possibility of acute compartment syndrome after childbirth. But how can they be aware of it if we don't educate our maternity care providers that such a complication *can* happen, irrespective of how rare it is? So, to answer your question, I want my case written up and published in a medical journal.'

My monologue was followed by a short silence. I looked at Dr White, who was looking pensively at the notes in front of him. Ms Arrow, staring intently into my eyes, remained silent. Dr Smith, as he had been through the whole meeting, was looking at his phone, not paying any attention to what I had just asked for. *Yeah, I know you think this is a waste of your precious time.* I ignored him.

There was silence in the room, but I was ready for a fight. I was prepared to fight for this.

'Yes. I'll contact the doctors involved and ask if they want to write it up,' replied Dr White.

I couldn't believe what I had just heard. Did he just agree to my massive request? Did he really say yes to having my case written up? I had walked into that room sure that they would never agree to this. 'Really?' I asked. 'You're really going to publish my case?'

'Well, we can't guarantee it will get accepted for publication, but I can promise I will do my best to have one of the doctors involved in your care write it up and submit it to a journal.'

Oh. My. Goodness. It happened. They agreed to write it up, even though it could potentially paint them in a bad light because they failed to diagnose the compartment syndrome on time. I was gobsmacked. And humbled.

Dr White's agreement to arrange for my case to be written—that in itself showed genuine acknowledgement of what had happened to me. Finally, they were not trying to cover up their mistakes. I told them I wanted it published in the Journal of Medical Case Reports because it allows the patient perspective to be included in the article. It was very important for me to contribute to the paper and include my perspective. I feel so many 'cases' are discussed clinically, and often the human side of it is left unacknowledged. Patients become 'cases' once they leave the hospital system, but patients live with the consequences of the care they received forever. These consequences are still very real and very recent for us as the patients, but the hospitals forget us because they see new patients every day. We become a distant memory. For me, having this doctor agree to write up my case to be published felt like another weight lifted off my shoulders.

I went home that day knowing that I had achieved my goal. I had fought so hard and for so long to be heard, be acknowledged, and have my wishes respected. Just like that, I no longer felt the need to continue with litigation. I felt no desire to continue fighting using lawyers. I didn't need lawyers anymore. My case was going to be written up.

I needed to heal now. That was my next journey. It was the attitude of the people in the room that day during the conciliation meeting (bar the orthopaedic guy) that changed it all for me. Their humility in accepting responsibility, acknowledging me for all that I am, not only a patient and complainant but also a clinician with specialised knowledge in the field, as well as their willingness to make amends and do something to improve maternity care on my behalf, was what allowed me to allow myself to let go. I had been heard, and now I had permission to breathe again.

Chapter 8

Months went by, and Elizabeth called to let me know that one of the doctors had agreed to write the paper, and one had already started working on it. I reminded Elizabeth of the agreement to have me involved in writing the paper so the 'patient perspective' could be included.

'I'll look into it and get back to you,' she said.

A few weeks later, Elizabeth called me again. This time, the news wasn't that great. The doctor who had agreed to write my paper had suddenly refused to continue once she heard I wanted to be involved.

'Why on earth doesn't she want to continue if I am involved?' I asked.

'I don't know, Sharon,' Elizabeth replied, clearly upset by this bump in the road. *'The doctor refused to give me a reason and said she is going to drop it completely now.'*

I remember the day so clearly. I was angry and articulated my feelings to Elizabeth. She was on my side, but she listed to me vent. Elizabeth was one of the few people who understood how important it was for me to have my case written up and published. She knew my reasons. And she was frustrated, too. After the mammoth wins I just had with the HCCC meeting, this felt like a giant leap backwards.

We talked about the possible reasons the doctor didn't want my involvement in writing the case, and after discussing a few possibilities, we both thought it could be due to fear of liability. Or maybe she feared any communication with me. It didn't matter anyway because the bad news was that no other doctor involved in my case wanted to touch the case report.

Elizabeth and I were both shocked and outraged at everyone's lack of interest in this. Didn't anyone want to improve medical care? Writing the case (and hopefully getting it published) would help other obstetricians in the same situation to quickly find information on ACS. Didn't anyone care about making a change?

But the reality was, and Elizabeth and I both knew, that no-one wanted their name associated with a case that didn't have a positive outcome. I had been doing my own research slowly and found several case reports on ACS within an obstetric context. All the cases I had found in the medical literature were cases where obstetricians had quickly identified the compartment syndrome and initiated limb-saving surgery for the new mother. Those published cases painted the doctors in a positive light for having identified the ACS quickly. Naturally, and understandably, it seemed that no-one here wanted to associate themselves with a case of delayed diagnosis. Elizabeth and I were both of the opinion that it shouldn't matter, however. The doctors shouldn't avoid publishing a case just because it had a bad outcome. The only way others would ever find out about the possibility of ACS as a rare but possible complication in childbirth was if there was more awareness on the topic.

'If no-one wants to write it up,' I said, 'then let me write my case report! I'll do it myself.'

'Really?' she asked, surprised that I would even consider doing this.

'Yes! I've been researching ACS ever since it happened to me. I have a collection of cases already, so why not?' I was dead serious. I just needed someone from the hospital to back me, someone who worked at the hospital and would be a co-author on the paper.

'Wait! I have an idea!' Elizabeth exclaimed excitedly. 'There's a new director of medical services who recently took on the position at the hospital. He's young, full of energy and enthusiasm, and he seems very passionate about improving health care. Let me talk to him and see if he can help us figure out a solution to our dilemma.'

I was too afraid to hope for a good outcome, but not too long went by before Elizabeth called me back with the exciting news.

'The new DMS wants to speak with you!' Elizabeth couldn't contain her excitement. 'He wants you to come in to the hospital to have a meeting with us both and discuss this!'

I couldn't believe my ears! *Wow!* I'd never heard of a DMS wanting to have a sit-down and chat with a complainant. Even Elizabeth was amazed by this. She was chatting away excitedly about all the possibilities now. She kept saying, 'He's young and innovative, and I like him. This one is going to make some change!'

I could feel it too.

A few weeks later, Elizabeth and I sat with the DMS in his office and discussed my case. The DMS was an eccentric, forward-thinking young man who seemed to have a positive outlook on things. He spoke with enthusiasm, and I instinctively liked him.

After listening to Elizabeth explain that none of the doctors wanted to write up my case, he expressed his genuine disappointment in the situation. 'I can't understand why no-one wanted to write it up,' he kept saying. 'But why? Why? It's a missed opportunity for education.'

I couldn't agree more.

The DMS sat pensively for a few minutes before asking, 'How can I help?'

A relieved smile appeared across Elizabeth's face.

Jumping at the opportunity, I said, 'I'd like to write up my own case report.' I explained that I had been searching the literature on ACS for the previous five years and accumulated a number of case reports. I wanted to have a go at putting it together myself.

'What a brilliant idea!' he exclaimed optimistically. 'And if no-one else in the hospital will agree to put their name on the paper, then I have no problem putting my own name on it for you.'

Oh, my heart! I was amazed by his kindness and understanding. I could have hugged him! He knew I would need the name of someone from the hospital to give my case report some clout. Since I am the patient in the case report, he knew I'd need either himself or one of the doctors who was involved in my care to support my publication. I was overwhelmed by this man's support of my mission.

Finally, Elizabeth and I had found someone who was on the same path that we were on, someone else who was in our lane, who was passionate about changing the healthcare system to improve patient care. He understood the importance of learning from mistakes to improve care.

'But *can* the patient author their own case report?' I asked them both. 'Would a journal actually publish it?'

Neither Elizabeth nor the DMS had ever heard of a patient who published their own medical case report, but 'Why not try?' replied the DMS. 'Who cares what others have or haven't done? Just because it hasn't been done before doesn't mean you can't be the first to try, does it?'

That night, I began writing my case report.

Life continued for me. I went about my daily life, and at night after my son was asleep, I got my laptop out and kept working on the case report.

One day, Elizabeth contacted me to tell me she had received a call from a TV show that was looking for stories of positive outcomes after hospitals had made mistakes. They had found more than enough negative stories already and now were on the hunt for a success story. After making calls to all the hospitals in the state, only Elizabeth was able to give the TV agent something positive. 'I thought you would be the perfect person for this show, Sharon.'

What an amazing opportunity to share my story on national TV, I thought. I was excited about the chance to educate other medical facilities on the importance of true, open disclosure and how to help patients move on with their lives.

It's okay to make mistakes. After all, hospitals are run by humans, and humans make errors. Healthcare workers don't go into fields caring fields like medicine, nursing, and midwifery with a plan to ruin someone's life. They're called 'caring professions' for a reason. But when mistakes are made, it's important for hospitals to get open disclosure right. It's about recognising and acknowledging the mistake, listening to the patient, and hearing the impact it has had on their life. It also includes offering a genuine apology and then providing a way forward. I sincerely believe the health care sector would see far less litigation against hospitals if only they learned how to perfect the art of open disclosure. Without open disclosure, people—patients who have suffered at the hands of the health care system—have a hard time moving on with their lives.

This is the message I wanted to get out to the hospitals.

I was excited about telling the world my story. Elizabeth asked for my permission to share my number with the TV station, and I consented.

Shortly after, Amy, the manager putting together the episode, called me to talk about my story. After having heard an overwhelming number of negative stories, Amy was blown away by my story of healing and repair and how the hospital had worked with me to facilitate change.

After getting all the details about my case and some documentation on the medical complication, Amy sent me two taxi vouchers to use to get to the studio and return home. The producers loved my story so much that they wanted me to be on the front panel and have a greater voice on the show instead of being seated in the audience. Amy asked for me to come in early to have my hair and makeup done. I was nervous but also very excited, so I went out and bought some new clothes to wear to the show.

Elizabeth and I prepared a lot over the weeks leading up to the recording of the episode. Elizabeth knew I was nervous, so she organised to come along to the studio to support me and help calm my nerves. I was grateful for Elizabeth. She had become more than just a patient representative at the hospital. She had been my advocate, my support, and my cheerleader in this mission I was on.

When the day arrived to go to the studio, dressed in my new clothes and nervous as ever, I was about to walk out the door when I received a call from Amy. At the last minute, the TV station's legal department had decided to not go ahead with the episode for fear of litigation. When the team had looked into the stories of other people due to appear on the show, it was discovered that the hospitals had not approved or confirmed the patient stories.

The episode didn't go ahead, but at least my fight to make change was heading in the right direction.

By this time, I was working full-time at a PHU, investigating cases of notifiable infectious diseases within the community, but it was a high-pressure job, and I was fed up with the regular on-call work that came with it. I was trying to raise my little boy on my own while paying rent in the inner-western suburbs of Sydney, all on a single income. I was also paying off part of a mortgage.

While I was still married, my son's father and I signed a contract to purchase land and build a house. However, not long after that, we separated. He didn't want anything to do with the mortgage, so I took it on myself. At the time, I thought it might be a good idea to own the property for my son's future, but I had the massive responsibility of also paying for it. I leased it out, but there was still a small margin left to pay that wasn't covered by the rental payments.

With everything on my plate, being on-call for the PHU made it too difficult to continue in that position. Having to be available to answer calls after hours—putting that in front of the needs of my little boy, who so desperately needed me to be an engaged and present mother—was too much for me. By this time, and not having taken annual leave from my job for two years, I was exhausted and on the verge of a mental breakdown. 'I need to take leave, and I need it now,' I desperately told my manager at work. 'I just can't keep going with the weight of the extra stress I'm carrying at the moment. I have six weeks of leave saved up, so can I please take it all now, or can I resign and have my leave paid out?'

I didn't care if I had to resign. I was desperate and mentally and physically exhausted. My manager, who knew the amount of stress I was under and what I had been going through, graciously arranged for me to take all of my six weeks of leave. That very day, I knew I needed to sell my house.

When I make a decision, I get on with it, so I immediately put the house on the market. It sold fairly quickly, leaving me with a small profit to figure out my finances. I paid both mine and my ex-husband's capital gains tax, bought a car, and took my little boy on a holiday to the Gold Coast. It was the last few months before he started kindergarten in 'big' school. We both absolutely loved having that time together. He was happy having me around more, which meant he didn't need to be in day care. And most of all, I could see he was happier that I was emotionally present in his life. And *I was happy*. It was just too good to leave this and go back to working full time again. I had missed out on so much of my son's early years, and I wasn't about to lose any more. After having those early years unceremoniously taken away from me, I wasn't about to let anything or anyone take any more of it from me.

While we were at the Gold Coast, I decided then and there that I wouldn't go back to working full-time. I called my manager the next day to let her know I wouldn't be coming back. My work did everything they could to keep me there, offering part-time and flexible hours, but regardless, the on-call would still be required. And I just was not going to be doing *that* anymore.

I resigned and lived off some of the profit I made with the sale of the house for the remaining few months of that year. I still had a deep, burning need to 'make up for lost time' before he was in school five days a week. To be there for him, to do the things I didn't get to do when he was a baby—I needed to restore that, if only in my own head. I know I could never achieve that because he will never be a little baby again, but that deep, unrelenting need was still there. Finally, though, I felt like I had been given the time, space, freedom, and money to at least try.

During the time that I was on leave from work, I had a lot of space to think about what I wanted to do.

Following my birth experience, I had several friends and colleagues reach out to me to share their own birth stories. They had experienced different complications, but the story was the same. Midwife, nurse, or doctor. Becomes the childbearing woman. Expected to rely on her own clinical knowledge during a time when she is transitioning to motherhood. Falls through the cracks of our maternity care system. Leaves the system traumatised and living with the consequences. For the women who had reached out and bravely shared their stories with me, I felt the need to be a voice and to affect change for them.

I made some calls, and before I knew it, I had written up a basic proposal for a PhD and submitted it to Western Sydney University. I was surprised and also somewhat amused when the university approved and accepted me into their PhD program. I only had masters' qualifications in coursework; I had not done honours or master's by research, so when I was accepted, I *knew* I was on the path destined for me. I knew in my heart and soul that this was my mission, and therefore, come rain, hail, or shine, no matter what, I was going to open the doors for women's voices to be heard.

My experience of being a childbearing woman became the catalyst for embarking on my PhD. I had to figure out how to survive financially for the following years of study, so I applied to teach at the university. I got to choose the days and hours I would work and the subject I would teach. It was the perfect job for me and meant that I could be there for my son, especially during his first year of school. This was so important to me. After all the issues I had when he was a baby, I was so desperate to make sure our connection as mother and son was solid and secure. I didn't want to miss out on anything—not even one school assembly. I scheduled my teaching around my son's school hours so I could drop him at school, go straight to work from

10 am – 2 pm, and still make it home in time for school pick up. Teaching tutorials at university and marking student assignments was the perfect set-up for me financially, and I could still be the mother I wanted to be—the mother my son needed me to be.

Chapter 9

In October 2016, shortly after I enrolled in my PhD, Elizabeth contacted me about the Patient Experience Symposium, a two-day event dedicated to sharing knowledge about improving the experiences of care for people.

The symposium for 2017 was due to be held in April and would be run by several large health agencies. Elizabeth suggested that we submit an abstract for presenting at the symposium. It would be a great platform to talk about what can happen when hospitals work together with their patients to affect change.

There was a lot of red tape involved in this process. Elizabeth had to submit proposals to the health district before we could even submit a draft. It was such a drama. I was overcome by astonishment at the hurdles we had to jump in order to do something positive. Eventually, Elizabeth received the green light from the district managers, and I set about putting an abstract together. To my utter surprise, our abstract was accepted, and we were allocated a slot to speak at the 2017 Patient Experience Symposium.

Before the Patient Experience Symposium came around, however, I had been asked to share my story at the Inaugural Innovations in Maternity Care Conference.

The 17 March 2017 was the first time I shared my birth story in a public forum.

I thought it would be easy. It had been over five years since the ACS, and I had written so much about it for clinical purposes, but I had never before spoken about my story in public. It was an incredibly difficult and emotional speech to deliver.

When I stood up at the podium, I saw an auditorium full of midwives staring at me, and I suddenly became afraid. I nearly ran out of the room before I opened my mouth. Yet I knew God had placed me there for a reason, and it was only by His grace and strength that I stood there and spoke the words that I had written down. I had been given a thirty-minute time slot, and for the whole thirty minutes, I spoke through tears. I spoke about my own birth experience, the importance of health care workers' attitudes, and the importance of listening to women in maternity care services. I spoke about birth trauma and the cost of not listening to women.

The midwives and maternity care managers in the auditorium were silently clinging to my every word. When I looked up, I could see tears streaming down some of their faces. I could hear the quiet crying of those whose hearts were touched by my words. As far as I could tell, it was a powerful and moving experience for them.

After I had spoken my last word, I was too emotional to stay for questions. I couldn't talk about it to anyone. I left straight away and ran to the car. I just wanted to go home.

Later that afternoon and for the following few days, I received many messages on Facebook from midwives who had been there and wanted to reach out and thank me for bravely sharing my story. They wanted me to know that my story had made them reflect and question their own practice. They wanted to make sure I knew I had left a positive impact on their lives. I was touched and overwhelmed.

It was *that* day, when I had the courage to look up in between words and saw the faces of the midwives, quietly listening and reacting to my words, tears streaming down some of their faces, that I finally realised the power of sharing my story.

When it finally came to speaking at the Patient Experience Symposium on 3rd May 2017, I felt a little more confident to speak in front of people. Elizabeth was going to stand up with me, so my nerves weren't quite as bad. Although Elizabeth was on annual leave at the time, she wasn't about to miss this big event. After all, *she* had worked so hard to effect change through my case.

Despite my confidence, when the time came to stand up and present my story, my nerves got the better of me, and I became emotional.

I opened my mouth, and as I spoke the words of the first sentence, my voice trembled and I couldn't go on.

Elizabeth held my hand and whispered encouragingly, 'You can do this, Sharon.'

I shook my head. 'I can't,' I whispered back. It was scary being in front of so many hospital managers who, to me, represented people like Ben Brander and Agnes Ding.

Elizabeth kindly started reading my speech for me. Hearing her speak my words out loud gave me courage. *No, this is my story, and I didn't come this far to chicken out.*

I dug deep, mustered up all the courage I could, and started reading my speech.

Strongly and fiercely, I spoke about the power of listening and open disclosure and how it really was the key to my healing. This is the speech I wrote and delivered at the 2017 Patient Experience Symposium:

> Introduction: Elizabeth
>
> How many of you are clinicians? *[About three-quarters of the auditorium raised their hands.]*
>
> How many of you have suffered an adverse or traumatic event in hospital yourself, or your family members? [*Several hands went up.*]
>
> How many have sent a letter of complaint to the hospital? [*Fewer hands were raised.*]
>
> Sharon's speech:
>
> In November 2011, within twenty-four hours of giving birth to my son, I developed an acute compartment syndrome in my right lower leg. A

rare complication following childbirth, but one that requires urgent decompressive surgery to prevent permanent damage and the need for amputation. Mine was not diagnosed definitively until day ten, although it had been queried by a neurologist at a much earlier stage.

As a direct result of the delayed diagnosis, I sustained permanent damage to the nerve and muscles in my leg. I lost many things because of this. There are too many things to talk about, but I lost my career in clinical midwifery and nursing; I lost my independence, my marriage. And most importantly, the impact this had on my ability to care for my baby in the first couple of years of motherhood was the most painful thing for me.

It is nothing short of a miracle that I didn't lose my leg, and I am thankful that I can walk and run and look after my son now. But I didn't always feel this way. I was angry for a long time. I wanted them to see just how much this had impacted my life and those close to me.

After I contacted Elizabeth for the first time to initiate the complaint process, I had a meeting with senior hospital managers a few months after I gave birth. I received an apology, but I felt that it was a defensive one. One which left me feeling like they were attempting to justify their staff's actions or lack of actions. One that wasn't sincere or empathetic to my pain and suffering. One that I felt failed to acknowledge the seriousness of the near miss that could have resulted in the loss of my leg.

I left that meeting feeling outraged. My thought processes revolved around 'they didn't listen to me then, and they're not listening to me now'. I was angry and frustrated. More like enraged.

I was angry that they just didn't seem to be able to acknowledge the depth of impact this had on me and the ongoing emotional and physical consequences that I've had to deal with. I was even more angry that they didn't seem to be able to see the seriousness of misdiagnosing an acute compartment syndrome. I was angry because the next mother who this happens to may not be as lucky as I was and could potentially lose a leg from a delayed diagnosis.

In sheer desperation to be heard and acknowledged, and feeling like I had no other option, I engaged a lawyer with the intent to take legal action against the hospital. I thought, *If they won't listen to me, then they'll have to listen to a lawyer.* All I wanted was to be heard.

I then began the extremely long, arduous, and painfully emotional process of relaying my birth trauma to the lawyers in a way that they could understand the depth of the impact this had had on my experience of motherhood. Contemplating litigation against the very hospital that trained me to be the midwife that I am was a foreign concept to me, one that I'd never entertained before and never thought I would do. But I felt betrayed and let down by the very system that I worked for and cared about and trusted so very much. *I was supposed to be 'one of them.' How could they have treated me like this?* was all I could think.

Over the next few years, there was communication between myself and the hospital, none of their replies ever deemed sufficient by my high standards that I now expected from them. I found arguments to every sentence in their letters to me, fuelling my anger and passion to make them see just what they had done, propelling me to go to great lengths to obtain policies, protocols, and guidelines that this hospital was required to adhere to.

Their inability to acknowledge the seriousness of misdiagnosing an acute compartment syndrome incapacitated my ability to allow myself to move forward because I didn't want anyone else to endure the emotional trauma that I've endured. My traumatic birth experience became my identity. It became all that I could talk about to anyone that would listen. Everything revolved around what happened, and each time I told my story, the bitterness within me grew stronger and stronger.

After tendon-lengthening surgery, when I was cleared to return to non-clinical work, I was seconded to work as a Patient Safety and Quality Manager. I learned a lot about how hospitals deal with incidents like mine. I gained more knowledge of how the system worked, and this empowered me to challenge the system, push for change, and make myself heard. I was finally empowered.

So, after writing to the HCCC, we finally had another meeting, what is called a 'conciliation meeting'. This was towards the end of 2015.

Four years later.

From the first call I made to Elizabeth, I have to say that she has been truly remarkable. I found in her someone who also believed in improving health care for the benefit of the population, someone who *heard* me and also felt the same way about this situation as I did. She advocated for me, and has done so, for so long. But what I really wanted was a true acknowledgement of what had happened from managers who were in positions of power to change things. I thought if they could see it the way I saw it, then they could do something about changing practice and making health care safer for patients.

I walked into that meeting ready for a fight, but also knowing that I at least had Elizabeth on my side. I was ready to argue every defensive statement they would throw my way, but I also felt like David getting ready to fight Goliath. In that room were doctors, Heads of Departments! They knew more than I did, they were more qualified than I was, and I was afraid that they would intimidate me into silence to get rid of the problem that I must have become for that hospital.

I spoke. Through tears, I explained how this impacted every aspect on my life, but mostly my experience of motherhood. I asked, 'How could all of this possibly happen?' I questioned them on how so many policies and protocols were breached.

After I had really ripped in to them, specifically the head of department for obstetrics, he simply responded in the most humble, kind, and caring manner. He said, 'You're right, Sharon.' He acknowledged everything I had pointed out and acknowledged that it shouldn't have happened. He agreed with me. And then he said sorry. It was a different apology to the first one I had received. It caught me off guard because of how he said it.

He wasn't even involved in my care, and yet his apology was genuine, and I could see that he truly meant it. And he wasn't speaking to me from his professional position as a doctor or even a manager. He spoke to me as a parent, empathising with me, trying to imagine what it would have been like if this had happened to his family. He acknowledged the depths of physical and emotional pain that I have endured as a result of the consequences of their care. He said sorry with no attempt to justify anything. It was an unguarded and unreserved apology.

When incidents like this occur, I think management staff within hospitals are afraid to apologise in this manner for fear of litigation. But it was that very way in which he apologised that made all the difference in the world to me. It was him and his response to me that led me to decide not to take legal action against the hospital. It was his response to me that allowed something in me to let go of the anger. I finally had received what I so desperately needed. For the first time, I felt like they had listened to me and that I'd truly been heard, acknowledged, and respected. No amount of money from suing the hospital would have achieved the same thing.

They asked me what I wanted. All I wanted was for my case report to be written up because, as a midwife, it is important for me that every single obstetrician and midwife knows that ACS *can* occur following childbirth, as rare as it may be. So, they agreed to start writing it up.

A short while after this, we ran into some unforeseen circumstances surrounding the case report. I was frustrated and could feel the amount of red tape that is there when trying to push boundaries. Elizabeth called me and said that there was a new director of medical services at the hospital who is very much focused on person-centred care and that he wanted to meet with me!

I was shocked because this is something that just doesn't happen. During this meeting, he listened and then asked me what he could do to help me! I was completely blown away. The way he saw it, not getting the case report out would be a missed opportunity for education and improving patient care.

So we planned to write the case report as a team, myself included, and we are currently in the process of it now. Ever since then, we've been working in partnership to challenge the system, break barriers, and push the boundaries to ultimately improve patient care. Speaking here today was one of Elizabeth's ideas. She's always been one to think outside the box. She was contacted last year by a TV show wanting patients with stories like mine. She wanted me to share my story on the show. Although the episode didn't go ahead, as far as I am aware, no other hospital was willing to speak to them.

While I may be justified in being angry because of the ongoing consequences of what happened, their response to me did more for me than words can describe. Their humility and sincerity in their attitude towards me, and their utter willingness to work with me to challenge the system to initiate change in ways that have probably never been manoeuvred between hospitals and complainants, is truly unique and was what allowed me to move forward, to take a step out of the place of my pain and use my experience to make maternity care safer for the mothers to come. Writing my own case report with their support was the very thing that led me to start my PhD in the experiences of pregnancy and childbirth when the birthing woman is a midwife.

I can talk about what happened now from a place of strength. But it came only after I felt that I had truly been heard, and my identity as not just a complainant but also a healthcare professional was acknowledged and validated by them. *That* is true person-centred care.

What I want to emphasise is that there is power in listening to patients. Although it took us five and a half years to get to this point, it doesn't need to. These three people—Elizabeth, the head of department for obstetrics, and the new director of medical services—should serve as examples for managers in other hospitals on how to provide true person-centred care when responding to patients who have suffered adverse outcome in hospital.

They remind me of the humanity within healthcare, the reasons why we first go into it, and they remind me that there are still people in positions of management who truly care. To those of you who feel you have been wronged or hurt by the way you were treated in hospital, I pray that you can find a way to allow yourself to let go and be healed. I found that through my faith in God, and that is what allowed me to forgive the very people in the hospital that I felt had wronged me. Because, after all, hospitals are simply made up of people. People who go into nursing, medicine, and midwifery because they want to make a difference—because they care. They never go in with the intention to cause harm or emotional trauma through their actions or behaviours.

There are too many broken and hurting people in this world. All you have to do is read the complaints that hospitals receive, and you will see it: *'They didn't listen to me.'* In the general birth trauma literature, you will find that between 20–48% of women around the world are reporting their birth experience as traumatic. And the majority of these births occurred in hospital.

And if you delve a little deeper into that literature, you'll find that the cause of so much of this trauma was related to the way they were treated and spoken to by their maternity care providers. All you have to do is go to a café and listen in on the conversations that mothers have with other mothers about their birth experience to see the truth in that. 'They didn't listen to me.' 'They didn't tell me what was happening.' 'I wasn't heard.' They will remember how they were treated; they

> will remember their trauma and suffer silently, possibly for the rest of their lives. Many won't speak up, and many won't persist for as long as I did to make themselves heard by the hospital.
>
> To those of you who are in this room with the power to make change happen, I want to say this: you have the power to start the healing process by acknowledging that the person has been wronged. By listening, by respecting them, and by letting them know that they have been heard.
>
> So, I'll leave you with this one request: please choose to be the change that this world so desperately needs.

I finished that speech to a loud round of applause. I was overwhelmed. I was happy. We did it! I felt a real sense of achievement.

The audience had a lot of questions for me. After that session, people approached and thanked me for sharing my story. I even had requests to speak at other venues! *What on earth was happening to me?* I went home that day on a high! What an achievement it was to be able to speak up there with Elizabeth and openly share what had happened, how we worked together to make a change.

The positive outcome from all of this highlights the importance of hospitals saying sorry when things go wrong and mistakes are made. A sincere and non-defensive apology, showing understanding and acknowledging the impact a mistake has had on the patient's life, can not only prevent litigation but, more importantly, bring healing and restoration for the patient. When hospitals and healthcare providers work alongside patients to achieve their desired outcomes, we look past the patient as a complainant and truly achieve person-centred care.

Meanwhile, my case report had been written and submitted to the journal. The peer-review process resulted in the editor asking for a little more information about the case, but at that time, Elizabeth had gone on leave indefinitely, and my life was rather chaotic, too. Unfortunately, the submission lapsed.

Never mind, I thought. I had found more articles on ACS following childbirth since I initially submitted it, so I refined my case report. It had been five years since the event, so I was able to include a section on my progress from my physiotherapist and my orthopaedic specialist.

This time, the paper looked much better, and it was ready for submission to the journal. Finally, on 4 May 2019, after all the co-authors had approved the final manuscript, I resubmitted my case report for publication.

I wanted the paper to be open access, so that meant I had to pay for it to be open access. It was far too much for me to afford from my personal finances, so in my cover letter to the journal editor, I asked for a fee exemption. In my cover letter, I disclosed that *I* am the patient in the case report and explained that we need more awareness of this complication within obstetrics. Having the report published as open access would serve that purpose. I wasn't too hopeful about getting an exemption, let alone getting the paper published, especially as I was the patient in the case report. I didn't know if the journal would accept it, but there was no harm in asking.

I waited and waited and waited some more for a response to my paper. A year went by, and I still hadn't heard about the outcome of my paper. I knew these things took time, but in my impatience, I anxiously emailed the editor of the journal. I really needed that paper published because it would give me some peace of mind that if another woman were in the same situation somewhere on the other side of the world, and if her obstetricians were unsure if it was or wasn't compartment syndrome, they could easily search and my case would come up, drawing attention to its possibility. My case report could potentially save a limb or life!

I checked the journal portal every day. Maybe twice or three times a day. Who am I kidding? I was obsessed. I just wanted it published. I didn't care about the impact factor of the journal—I just wanted it published.

Eventually, on 9 July 2020, I received the long-awaited news that my paper had been peer-reviewed, and not only did it *not* require any changes, but it was *accepted for publication!*

And I got the fee exemption I had asked for!

I was elated. Excitement, gratitude, and an overwhelming flood of relief came over me. I was over the moon.

I can't believe how long it took, but finally, I had an acknowledgement of the reality of this rare but extremely serious limb- and life-threatening complication following childbirth. I felt validated. *My story is real.* It has been a roller coaster of a ride to get to this point, but I got there. By the grace of God, I got there.

If this paper could raise awareness and educate maternity care providers about this potential complication in obstetrics, if it can prevent just one other woman from a delayed diagnosis or limb amputation and the subsequent trauma of it all, all of what I have been through and fought for would be worth it. I can't prevent anyone from having ACS, but I can help by making sure maternity care providers are educated and aware that it can happen.

I had finally been given the closure I had been looking for all these years.

What a journey it had been.

Chapter 10

Acute compartment syndrome following childbirth is rare.

But birth trauma is not.

Over the years since my compartment syndrome, there have been many signs that I had PTSD. These signs, which I refused to acknowledge until recently, were clear as daylight to everyone around me—but not myself. Either consciously or subconsciously, I ignored these signs, sweeping them under the rug until one day when my mind spiralled out of control.

The day my son was rushed to hospital and ended up having emergency surgery was the day of my unravelling. I remember how the doctors took my son into the operating theatres and prepared me for what would happen—but nothing prepared me for the vacant look in his eyes when the anaesthetic settled into him. I freaked out in the operating theatres and begged the doctors to give him back to me alive and safe. 'He's my everything, my only child,' I cried. 'You have to promise to give him back.'

Thankfully, I *did* get my boy back, alive and safe. He was transferred to the paediatric ward for the night, and I stayed by his side the whole time. I tried to sleep in the fold-out chair next to his bed, but instead, I was anxiously watching the rise and fall of his chest, making sure he was alive. I couldn't allow myself to sleep. My mind was spiralling out of control. Without realising it, I was waiting for the ten-hour post-op mark because it was about then that the compartment syndrome began in my leg. I had to wait to make sure nothing happened to my baby. Fortunately, the remainder of the night went smoothly and we had no adverse outcomes, but this was the state of my mind at the time.

He was discharged the next day and recovered well.

But my mental well-being was deteriorating.

Being in hospital that night and watching my son go through an emergency operation was a major trigger for me. That night was the start of some serious flashbacks. I had panic attacks and was waking up with night sweats, having nightmares that my leg was raging red and blowing up again. Even if I had the slightest pain in one of my legs, I couldn't allow myself to sleep because I was terrified that I would wake up with acute compartment syndrome brewing again. These symptoms continued until I eventually cracked. I had a mental breakdown.

I *finally* took myself to a GP, who prescribed lorazepam to calm my nerves and referred me to a psychiatrist. After deliberating some more about whether I should actually see a psychiatrist or not, I eventually *did* go. I was immediately diagnosed with severe chronic PTSD and commenced on duloxetine. I also (finally) started seeing a psychologist to begin the journey of acknowledging and dealing with my birth trauma.

On 12 June 2019, the day I was officially diagnosed with PTSD, I wrote the following entry in my journal:

> Today, I was finally diagnosed with chronic PTSD relating to the events that took place hours after the birth of my son. It's taken seven and a half years to have the courage to see a psychiatrist. My healthcare providers have been trying to get me to see a psychiatrist ever since this happened, but I have resisted for so long.
>
> I knew I had PTSD. It was obvious. But I just didn't want to go and see anyone. Over the years, certain events have triggered my severe reactions. When I had the tendon-lengthening surgery, I thought I could feel my leg swelling under the bandage. The rational part of my brain knew that it wasn't, but the paranoid part fully believed it was blowing up inside there. I was scared of getting another compartment syndrome, but then again, there was that part of me that didn't want to cause a fuss and be 'that' annoying patient. I wanted to be the perfect patient after all the drama of being inside a hospital for fifteen days after giving birth and seeing how one of my midwives reacted to me, knowing how she complained about me in

the handover room. This time, I wanted to be the patient that no-one could complain about. After all, I am a perfectionist. My need for perfectionism has slowly tamed itself the longer I have been a mother, but the perfectionist's ugly head rears itself sometimes. I remember before the tendon-lengthening surgery, I put on a brave face the whole time until my surgeon asked me if I had any questions, and I crumbled into tears, asking him if this was going to happen again. He reassured me and promised me it would not.

Then there were the two pregnancies I had after the birth of my son. Although I desperately wanted to have another baby, 99% of me just freaked out about another compartment syndrome happening again. I became so scared and worried about losing my ability to be a mother to this new child if I had another untreated compartment syndrome, it was the only thing going through my mind. I was devastated when I miscarried, but there was relief, too. Because there was no way in the world I would survive another ACS and what it would have meant to go through all of that rubbish again. I couldn't bear to even think of having to lose my independence again, lose those early years of motherhood again, be a burden to everyone around me again, and go through all of it. I just couldn't.

One of my miscarriages ended up in a dilatation and curettage in the operating theatres because although my baby died inside me, my body didn't expel the foetus. I had to go under anaesthetic and have my baby removed. Shortly after that, I had to have another dilatation and curettage to investigate the reasons for having multiple miscarriages.

Before each dilatation and curettage, I freaked out on the inside about having my legs in stirrups—in the lithotomy position—because that is a known risk factor for developing ACS. My clinical brain knew that the risk for ACS is dependent on the length of time my legs are in the lithotomy position, but my PTSD brain wasn't able to reconcile any of that when it came to my absolute fear of ACS occurring again.

Then there was the surgery I needed in 2016 to correct a deviated septum (really crooked cartilage in my nose). I wasn't able to breathe properly, so it was finally time to get this fixed. At that time, I hadn't had a panic attack in eight months. I had even just enrolled in a PhD, and I was fine. I had been totally and completely fine. And I believed that.

Then the night before the nose surgery, I flipped out and almost cancelled it. I was driving myself mad that night, worrying about developing ACS after the surgery. I called a friend, who talked me through it and calmed me down. But the next morning, while waiting in the waiting room to be taken into the operating theatre, I was so anxious that I cried there, pacing the room in a total fluster in front of everyone else waiting to be taken in for their operations. In the pre-op room, when they inserted the cannula into the vein of my hand and asked me my name and date of birth for the tenth time, I became hysterical again. The surgeon didn't know how to respond to me and said, 'I've never seen someone quite so anxious before such a simple procedure.'

In the hysteria triggered by being in that pre-op room again, taking my mind back to being in the pre-op room just before I had the caesarean, I couldn't care less what he thought of me. 'Promise me,' I demanded through tears, 'that you will keep an eye on my leg.'

'What do you mean?' he replied, confused. 'I'm not going anywhere near your leg.'

'I *know* that, but for goodness' sake, can you just tell me you won't let anything happen to my leg? I *need* you to say that you won't let anything happen to my leg; otherwise, you can't take me into that operating theatre.' I was a disaster.

The poor man looked bewildered, unable to understand where this fear was coming from. So I told him what had happened to me, and he finally understood my reactions.

When I woke up after the operation, the first thing I asked was, 'Is my leg there?' I didn't care about my nose. I didn't care how that operation went. I cared only about my leg.

Throughout the years, I would be 'fine' for a while. Sometimes, months would go by between panic attacks. But whenever I felt even the slightest pain in either of my legs, my thoughts went straight to ACS. It was completely irrational to the rational mind, but to the PTSD mind, it made perfect sense. If my leg was sore at night, I simply would not sleep. I couldn't sleep. I was too terrified to sleep. Why? Because of how the pain progressed in the middle of the night when the ACS happened. It started off with a dull ache and slowly progressed to the most horrendous pain I have ever experienced in my entire life.

Still, I had never seen a psychologist about my birth trauma. I can give you a million reasons why I didn't go to see anyone for help. And they all made sense to me at the time. *I don't need help. I'm fine. I can do this. I'm strong. I don't have time to see a psychologist.*

Life went on. My body started to compensate for the physical deficits caused by the permanent damage to my right leg. I lived in physical pain every day, and still do, but I just had to get on with it ...

And get on with I did, until my son's surgery, when my carefully compartmentalised headspace came crumbling down around me. When he went into the theatre, I walked in there with him. Seeing the big, bright lights above the operating table took me straight back to being under those lights when they did the caesarean on me.

Not too long after that, my son had to have another surgery on his foot, and I was retraumatised being in there. He wasn't coping, too. He was hungry because he had been fasting before the operation. He was screaming for food in the theatres. I held it all together in front of him, but the moment he was inside the operating room, all my emotions came out. I could feel I was emotionally slipping, barely holding it together. To make matters worse, I also had to have another operation. Within two months, we had been in hospital three times. It was freak-out central in my head. This time, the surgeon and anaesthetist knew my history, were both a lot more understanding about my fears, and promised me I wouldn't be in stirrups for too long.

I came out fine, but my head was still a mess to the point where I had lost my ability to empathise. I remember another woman in my church had just had a baby and suffered a horrible two-litre post-partum haemorrhage. Listening to her story sent my mind spinning, and

> I found myself needing to excuse myself from listening anymore.
>
> *What the heck has happened to me? Have I lost my ability to empathise? What have I become?* I knew I needed to get my head sorted out. I was normally an empathetic and compassionate person, especially when it came to other women's birth experiences. I just couldn't handle it now. Finally, I knew that if I was going to be of any use in giving a voice to the women I was doing this PhD for, I had to sort myself out so that I could actually be of use and service to others.
>
> I finally went to see a GP, who started me on medications for anxiety and what he said was postnatal depression ... seven years on. My national survey for my PhD was soon due to be released, and I knew I couldn't possibly read about other women's birth stories. The GP ordered six months of urgent leave to get help and get myself back together. I was sent to crisis care with a psychologist and started treatment with a psychiatrist who specialised in PTSD in healthcare workers.

I often ask myself why I didn't go to get help much earlier. Why had I put it off for so long? On reflection, I supposed one of the biggest reasons was because I didn't want to be a statistic. But I can't explain to you why I didn't want to be a statistic.

I didn't want to acknowledge that something was wrong. Somehow, it made me foolishly think I was weak. Actually, for the first few years, I kept telling myself I was okay. I busied myself studying and undertaking more degrees. I have several unfinished degrees! The psychologist figured out why I kept throwing my mind into anything *but* dealing with my issues. She said, 'Many people turn to drugs and alcohol to cope with life, but you somehow turned to collecting degrees as your coping mechanism.'

Studying kept my mind busy and distracted me from the reality of what was going on. It didn't give me the time and space to delve into my pain and deal with it. Studying became my escape.

Although I do love learning, I no longer use studying as an escape. I have now dealt with many of my demons and come to peace with having PTSD. My medication helps me have nightmare-free sleeps and has significantly reduced the flashbacks, but I have to take it every day without fail. While I would one day love to be able to live a life without needing the help of medications, for now, I need it, and I am okay with that.

Chapter 11

Dear maternity care providers,

In the few short years I worked as a midwife, I worked in one low-risk hospital and two tertiary referral hospitals. I somehow always ended up looking after women who had all the crazy, complicated emergency births. It used to drive me mad that I never got to be involved in as many calm, natural births as I did crash caesareans or neonatal resuscitations. Actually, the first birth I ever attended as a student midwife was a caesarean section, which happened to be in the same operating theatres in which doctors lifted my own baby out of me. I remember being terrified as a student waiting to receive the baby in theatres.

And I was terrified as the woman being wheeled into the operating theatres, where I knew exactly what they were going to do to me. I knew how they would cut me open and pull my muscles apart, and I knew the blood bath that my stomach would become. I knew because I had seen it all too often and watched as the obstetrician took the baby out of the woman's uterus. But for the first time, *I* was that woman, and someone else was the midwife watching *my* uterus being cut open.

When I, a midwife, became a childbearing woman, I needed you to remember that I was a woman, too. I had a unique set of knowledge and skills that made me a little different from other women, but I also needed the space and freedom to be the birthing woman and not the professional midwife. I needed to be able to trust you and be allowed to let go and give birth without fear of judgment for asking a seemingly silly question that you expect me, as a midwife, to know the answer to.

I was feeling all the same feelings of new motherhood—fear, worry, and anxiety.

My anxiety levels were heightened because of all the things I knew could go wrong. I had the same pregnancy and new mamma hormones coursing through my veins as the mother in the bed next door to me.

When I was the childbearing woman, in that vulnerable state, I couldn't think in two minds. I couldn't be the clinician and the new mother at the same time. You wouldn't expect a lawyer to prepare a court case in those days of new motherhood, so why would you expect me to think with my clinical brain when I was going through such an important milestone in my life? I was just as vulnerable as any other mother who comes to you for maternity care. I was just as afraid and overwhelmed and exhausted as the next woman. Why did you expect me to just know to get on with breastfeeding and all these things when I had never done it before? Yes, I'd supported new mothers through these things, but that was in the role of a maternity care provider, in our work mode. I was not in that mode when I was becoming a new mother, yet I was expected to be.

When I was in that vulnerable position as a 'patient', you forced me to rely on my own professional knowledge to make your job easier. It made it harder for me to speak up and demand attention because I was afraid of how you would view me, afraid that you would complain about me at the handover meetings. But I already *knew* you were complaining about me.

It disempowered me.

I was afraid to make a fuss and call for help or press the buzzer because I knew how busy and overworked you were. Because I, too, was busy and overworked when I was working in your shoes.

I didn't want to be a troublemaker when I knew you had so much to do and so many other mums needed your support, too.

When my leg started to hurt, I wasn't complaining of pain because I wanted to stay in hospital for fifteen days and almost lose my leg. I wasn't complaining because I wanted to be bed-bound and not care for my son. I wasn't complaining because I wanted to bother you and add work to your already busy shift. I was complaining *because I was in agonising pain.*

But I didn't want to overplay things because I knew that you would roll your eyes and complain about me to your colleagues: 'That troublemaker over in bed two is complaining about her leg again.' I was scared to speak up and demand that you get me some medical help now because I was also worried that I was overthinking and exaggerating things. I was scared that you would say, 'She's making a big deal out of nothing.'

To the doctor who delivered my diagnosis: I remember when you came into my room in the middle of the night to tell me I had acute compartment syndrome, according to the scans. You asked me if I was nurse-trained. When I replied, 'Yes,' you said, 'You probably know more about it than I do.' And the reality was that I probably did know more about it than you did. I should have been taken to the operating theatres immediately or had the surgeons see me then and there, but instead, you said the surgical team would see me the next morning. That told me you had no idea how serious acute compartment syndrome is. I asked you a ridiculous question: 'Will my leg burst open between now and then?' The silliness of that question is not lost on me, but it should have told you how petrified I was. Clinically, I knew this wouldn't happen; I knew the ACS would crush my arteries and nerves. But in my terrified state, I was panicking. I should have spoken up and demanded that you do something then and there. I mean, you don't just deliver such a serious limb- and life-threatening diagnosis in the middle of the night and leave the patient to sit and wonder on their own, especially when the patient has some clinical knowledge of the gravity of the diagnosis.

I wanted to say something to make you do more than just waltz off out of there. But then my clinical mind started getting paranoid, and I questioned myself.

Maybe I'm overreacting? Maybe I don't know as much as I do. They're doctors; they know what they're doing. Maybe there's something I don't know about this, and that's why they are not rushing to get me urgent surgical intervention. So I just let you walk out of my room because I didn't want to make a fuss and be seen as stupid for not knowing something that I should have known as a midwife. You left me there to panic about my situation with my mum, who also didn't know what was going on. You left me there, alone in my fears and worries, and did absolutely nothing to reassure me that I was going to be okay and that I wouldn't lose my leg. You knew I was scared I would lose my leg, but you did nothing to console me. I was scared and alone in a hospital that I thought I was safe in, a medical system that I worked for and believed in. *Is this how other women feel when they are in our maternity care system?*

In my experience as the birthing woman, I was stuck somewhere between the identity of patient and health professional but never acknowledged as either. This is how birth trauma turned me, a midwife, into a disempowered and vulnerable 'patient' who had lost agency. This is how I fell through the cracks.

Falling through the cracks of our maternity care system led me to the silent and lonely struggle with postnatal depression and PTSD, marring my experience of motherhood.

Chapter 12

Everything that happened to me and the emotional pain I endured—these are not just the scars of undiagnosed and untreated ACS. These are the deep scars caused by a healthcare system that failed to treat me as a birthing woman—*a person.*

It is important, however, to highlight that the majority of my care providers were wonderful. The midwife who looked after me during labour went over and above to stay with me during my very long labour, all the way until I was taken back to the postnatal ward after the caesarean. She advocated for me during labour and created a safe place for me to labour in. She knew what I wanted, and I trusted her judgment. When she finally suggested an epidural, I trusted her. Two hours after the epidural, she told me that my cervix had thickened, and after many hours of labour, I knew we had to do the caesarean.

I am not traumatised by the caesarean or by the fact that I could not have a normal vaginal birth. I received the best care from my midwife during my labour. I trusted her, I felt safe with her, my identity as a professional midwife was acknowledged and respected, and I was able to let go and fully be the labouring woman in her care. I am forever grateful for her. Many of the midwives who cared for me after the acute stage of compartment syndrome were incredibly caring. Even some of the obstetric registrars were kind and caring; one obstetrician came to check in on me when she was rostered to work in the antenatal clinic for the day!

While I am eternally grateful for those who showed me genuine kindness, care, and empathy, the impact of the delayed diagnosis on my life and the depth of pain I have experienced have been enormous, and words on paper just cannot do it justice. I have been on a long and tumultuous journey, and God has blessed me and continues to strengthen me.

Nothing could have prevented me from developing compartment syndrome, but listening to me, believing me, and taking me seriously could have changed the outcome of the complication. I could have been seen earlier by specialists who could have performed surgery sooner and prevented the permanent functional restrictions and pain I now live with.

The attitude of maternity care providers when providing care for birthing women is so important and can have long-lasting consequences. As maternity care providers, the way we talk about women makes a big difference. I know the midwife who 'looked after' me that first day was complaining about me to the other midwives in the handover room. I *knew* it in my gut. I remember telling another midwife that I no longer wanted that particular one looking after me. I said, 'I bet she's always whinging about me in handover.' This midwife, with a despondent look on her face, said, 'Yes, she is.' But I didn't need her to confirm that to me. I already knew it was happening. I knew because I am guilty of having done the same thing when I was frustrated about the number of times some women had rung the buzzer all night long on a shift. When I couldn't sit down for more than five minutes before another buzzer went off, I remember wondering why they didn't want to get up and do things for themselves. I remember thinking those horrible things. It is common to vent about patients in handover to colleagues. There is a culture within health care, particularly midwifery, to vent or complain about the women we care for to our colleagues during handover.

But let me tell you something. That culture and attitude have a cost.

Not listening to women has a cost.

I lost so many things that were precious to me as a direct result of not being listened to.

The last shift I worked before going on maternity leave was my last ever shift as a clinical midwife. And I grieve the loss of that. A lot.

I can't even begin to explain how this affected my marriage. The pressure was enormous. We never really got the chance to adjust to the role changes under normal circumstances. Eventually, the pressure from all of this significantly contributed to the end of my marriage. I never thought the circumstances and consequences of childbirth could entrench themselves so deeply that it could destroy precious relationships. I never thought I'd become a single mother and have to raise my son on my own.

For me, it wasn't the agonising pain of compartment syndrome or even the loss of my career or my marriage, as painful as it all was. The physical consequences that affected my ability to carry my son and provide care for him, challenging my identity as his mother, were what destroyed me the most. I missed out on all of that.

I remember working night shifts on the postnatal wards, putting other women's babies to sleep, rocking them in my arms, pacing corridors with them, longing for a time when it would be my own baby that I was putting back to sleep in my arms, against my chest. But when that time came, it wasn't me who did that for my child. I had to watch others comfort and reassure my baby. Even though it was my own family, it still wasn't *me*, his mother, who attended to his needs. And it grieves me and causes so much heartache that I couldn't. This is the loss that I *still* have a hard time coming to terms with.

With everything that happened, *that* is the thing that still causes me so much heartache. *That* is the thing that I still have a hard time dealing with and coming to terms with. And I will never get that back.

I felt like those early years of motherhood were taken away from me simply because they didn't listen to me.

When I was wearing my work uniform and work badge, what I said mattered. My words carried weight. I had the power to make things happen. But the moment I was the birthing woman in that bed, wearing a patient gown instead of my work uniform—suddenly I was simply a bed number. Nothing I said mattered or carried any weight.

Even with my knowledge and background in midwifery, with them knowing that I was a midwife—because I had done my midwifery training at that very hospital, had worked with those midwives and doctors—I felt like I wasn't listened to.

How much harder is it for other women? Despite being a midwife, I still felt so vulnerable and disempowered, my life in the hands of these healthcare workers, some of whom I felt didn't truly care or want to listen to me. If it was that hard for me, then how hard must it be for the multitudes of women who walk through the doors of our maternity services to be listened to, to be heard, to be believed in and taken seriously?

My dear friends and colleagues in maternity care, when we as maternity care providers don't listen, we strip a woman of her power and identity. When we don't take her seriously, there is a cost.

When you complain about her in the handover room, you colour the other midwives' and doctors' perceptions of that woman and could potentially affect the rest of her care. When you do that, you take away her human right to unbiased, unprejudiced, woman-centred care. With shame, I admit that I am guilty of having done this very thing to women when I worked as a midwife. But I have also felt the impact of this. That is the reason I am sharing my experience with you. When that midwife complained about me to everyone else, it affected how seriously the others took my complaints of pain. 'She's complaining about her leg again,' is what some doctors had been saying about me. I know that because a doctor who was involved in my care told me what she had heard from other medical teams who were also involved in my care.

Every time that midwife came in to answer my buzzer, she was sighing, rushing in to cancel the buzzer, displaying all the body language of frustration. I could tell. I could read body language just like many other women who come in and watch the way we provide care for them. And I knew that language well because I remembered, with guilt and shame, the times during some of my own busy shifts when I had behaved just like that.

Most of you will probably never see acute compartment syndrome in a postpartum woman, and I hope you never will. But, my friends and colleagues, you will see a woman who presses the buzzer because her pain relief isn't working, because she can't get up and pick up her baby, because it's too painful and hard to walk to the bathroom, because she is struggling to come to terms with how her labour turned out and she doesn't know how to cope with it all, and suddenly she has a little human being relying on her for everything. And she is exhausted. When she presses that buzzer, she needs you. She needs you to be her kind, caring, and compassionate care provider. And how you walk into that room to answer that buzzer really matters. It might just be another shift to you, but that woman will remember the way you walked in there and the way you responded to her, probably for the rest of her life. Childbirth is a sacred and precious moment, and women remember how they felt and how they were treated.

And they will remember for a very long time.

In your position, my dear friends and colleagues in maternity care, I urge you to acknowledge and understand the power that you hold. You have so much power over the lives of childbearing women, and it is easy to take that for granted. I know because I was once the midwife providing care to birthing women, and I know how easy it is to forget this. Please remember that you hold all the power to either make or break her.

And you also have the power to start the healing process for her.

For me, it came four years later when I was finally heard by the managers of that hospital. They finally listened and acknowledged the impact the delayed diagnosis had on my life. I had challenged the system and kept pushing all these years until I was heard. And finally, something changed for me. I want to honour and express my deepest and most sincere gratitude to those who truly listened to me and acknowledged me as not just as a 'complainant', but also as a healthcare professional with specific knowledge and experience that enabled me to understand the healthcare system in a different way. There is great power in listening. It was only when I felt that they listened to me and their attitude toward me had changed that I was really able to allow myself to truly start to heal from the emotional trauma that had been the previous few years of my life. I was finally able to take a step out of the place of my pain and start doing something positive from all of this.

However, the sad thing is that it shouldn't have taken that long to be heard. It should have happened when I was a birthing woman in that hospital bed of that postnatal ward.

I had to push for change myself, and it was only after I worked at the Patient Safety and Quality Unit, after I learned how to conduct clinical investigations of incidents that occurred in hospital and how hospitals deal with incidents, that I was able to do something to force change. Through my experience at the PSQU, I gained even more insider knowledge of how the healthcare system worked, and therefore I was empowered to challenge the system, push for change, and finally make myself heard.

But many women who have had negative or traumatic experiences in our maternity services may not do the same thing. Many wouldn't know where to begin, and many may be disempowered because of what happened to them. And many won't persist for as long as I did.

What about the women who experience traumatic births in our hospitals and don't know how to deal with it and can't heal and move forward? They may forever feel that they weren't heard at such a crucial time in their lives. It is such a disempowering feeling, and many will live with their birth trauma forever.

Even as a midwife and having worked within the system, it was still so hard for me to speak up and have a say in the care I received. How much harder must it be for others who don't have the same insider knowledge?

I know how fortunate I am to still have my leg, and it is nothing but the grace of God that allows me to get through each day without falling back into the place of my pain. And my faith, although it is only the size of a mustard seed at times, is what allows me to keep going and continue moving forward.

It is because this happened to me that I can write about this, not as a midwife but as a birthing woman, and speak for the many other women who come through the doors of our maternity services and need you, my dear friends and colleagues, to reconsider how you provide care to them.

A nurse I know still remembers overhearing what her midwife said about her to another midwife, just outside the door of the labour room: 'That psycho problem in there ... and she's a bloody nurse.' My dear friends and colleagues, a throwaway sentence like that when you are tired on a shift might mean nothing to you, but it can stay with someone for a very long time. That stuck with her for five years until she had intensive therapy to come out of her trauma.

My story is just one of the many other stories of birth trauma. Too many women around the world are reporting their birth experience as traumatic, and the ongoing impact of birth trauma is what maternity care providers don't see after women are discharged from their care. The way their lives are impacted is not captured in the hospital birth and medical records.

Birth trauma is a silent public health emergency that needs to be addressed. Birth trauma and its impact is a very real and serious problem. It can impact every part of a woman's life. We need to start seeing the bigger picture of birth trauma and the impact it has on society. It can damage relationships, leading to relationship breakdown; often, it will leave a woman to raise children on her own.

Birth trauma isn't solely about physically traumatic births. The interactions with maternity caregivers play a big role in how women perceive their birth experience. The way women are treated, including the way they were spoken to and if they are dismissed or not listened to, impacts on whether they consider their birth experience traumatic.

There is something seriously wrong with the way we provide maternity care to women, and it is time we address this silent public health emergency. Birth trauma silently impacts women's lives, and when it impacts women, it has an impact on society. I am acutely aware that the notion of birth trauma being only a woman's issue is a popular thought, but I want to challenge that idea. Birth trauma is *not* just a woman's issue. It is not just a mother's issue.

Birth trauma is society's issue, and we need to address this. Now. Before it becomes a problem for the next generation of childbearing women.

My dear friends and colleagues in maternity care, what you do, what you say, and how you say it has a cost. But you also have the privilege of having access to such a sacred and special time of a woman and her family's life. To be a maternity care provider is a privilege and an honour, and it should be treated as such. You have the power to allow a woman to perceive her transition into motherhood as a positive experience. Even when things don't go to plan, the way you treat her can make all the difference in the world to her. You have the power to make or break her. So please choose to make her.

My birth experience changed the course of my life. It almost broke me completely, but it didn't. Instead, I have fought tooth and nail and chosen to let it make me. Even though I sometimes do get emotional about it, I am not stuck in the place of my pain anymore. My son's fifth birthday was the first time I didn't cry with the memory of what happened when he was born. It was the first time I saw what happened to me in a positive light. It was the first time I began to be grateful for the opportunity that this experience has opened up for me. Because of that, I can talk and write about this today, be a voice for the multitudes of women who come through the doors of our maternity services each and every day, and remind you, my dear friends and colleagues, that they need you.

They need you to care for them.

They need you to listen to them.

And they need you to believe in them.

I don't want anyone else to walk through what I have had to endure. It has been extremely difficult for me to revisit my old journal entries about my experience, to go back to a place where I once was and relive those painful emotions. But I believe we get our greatest joys and success from the place of our deepest pain. So if my story can get your attention and cause you to take birth trauma seriously, if my story can lead maternity care providers to reflect on their own clinical practice and listen to the women they care for, to *really listen* and respect what they have to say, if my story can improve maternity care for others and help prevent traumatic birthing experiences for childbearing women, then every ounce of physical trauma and pain I have endured and still experience on a daily basis, and every tear that I have cried, and every aspect of motherhood that was robbed from me as a new mother, and every scar that has developed, would have been worth it all.

Epilogue

I started documenting my story from the very beginning when the midwifery educator who had trained me as a student came to visit me in hospital and told me quietly to 'write it down'. When I was a midwifery student under her guidance, she would always say to me and my colleagues, 'Document it all.' This was her mantra, and that mantra stuck with me.

I wrote, never once thinking the events that took place after I gave birth would change my life so drastically. Throughout the years, I kept writing, journaling about my experience, emailing hospital managers and lawyers, and writing for conference presentations. These pieces of writing have become the contents of this book.

Ten years have gone by since I gave birth to my son and developed ACS. I have had a very full, emotional, and wonderful ten years since I became a mother.

I was broken and shattered. My birth trauma caused my world to crumble down around me. The trauma engulfed me and swiftly took away so much that was dear to me. When I got married at the age of twenty-two, I never once thought I would one day become a single mother.

While that phase of my life was tough, those five years of single motherhood were an abundance of blessings in disguise. I got five solid years with my son, just he and I. I worked hard, but I also played hard. We went on holidays together, even overseas on our own. We spent time—*real* time—together. We connected in a way that I probably never would have been able to if my birth had gone according to *my* plan. I got time to focus on him and motherhood, and it was good. And it *is* good. Today we are thick as thieves!

Despite the past, my son's dad and I are friends, and we will always work together to do what is best for the child we brought into this world together. My son is never restricted from spending time with his dad, stepmother, and stepsisters. They regularly have weekends together and talk on the phone freely.

Throughout the last ten years, I have questioned my faith frequently. Having been raised a Christian, as the eldest child of a pastor, I couldn't understand what had happened to my life. I fought to cling to what I knew of God and what I had been taught. I used to get angry at God and question His promises, which I was *supposed* to believe in.

But God has been gracious and faithful to me. And just as promised, He restores what the locusts have eaten (Joel 2:25–27).

I have since met the love of my life and am happily remarried. Ronen is the most wonderful, kind-hearted, caring, generous, and loving man on this planet. Marrying

Ronen has also given me two beautiful stepchildren. Ronen loves me and our three children fiercely, and he does anything and everything for us. His values about parenthood and putting our children first aligns with mine, and we work well as a team.

Because of his love and generosity, I have been blessed with the freedom to focus on what my heart wants to do—to be a mother, to finish my PhD, and to put my energy into working towards ending birth trauma for others.

I have scars. But my heart is full.

Scars

The Oxford Advanced Learners Dictionary defines a *scar* as:

A. a mark that is left on the skin after a wound has healed
B. a permanent feeling of great sadness or mental pain that a person is left with after an unpleasant experience
C. something unpleasant or ugly that spoils the appearance or public image of something.

My journey has left me with many scars, both physically and emotionally. Some of these scars are minor, but some run deep and are etched permanently within the crevices of my psyche.

I used to think that scars are ugly, but life has taught me to appreciate my scars. By the grace of God, my battle scars have turned into scars of gold.

And if my journey is proof of anything, it's that it *is* possible to turn your scars to gold.

My Recommendations—Conscious Maternity Care

For all of you who are maternity care providers, I would like to suggest a new, gentler way of providing care—Conscious Maternity Care.

I think we can make a big difference in the way women perceive their birth experience by consciously making little changes in our approach to care. I want to make some recommendations that I think will help you to better provide conscious maternity care:

1. Be aware of your own biases, beliefs, fears, and concerns. For example, if you fear a potential complication in a certain situation, which may well have arisen from your experience in witnessing such complications, be conscious that the women you care for may not share those same fears as you. Be mindful not to project that fear onto the women you care for.
2. Your words matter. Every little word you speak out loud is heard, absorbed, and internalised by the women you care for. You will likely forget your throwaway comments, but be conscious that the women you care for *will* remember.
3. Mind your body language. This matters a lot. Even if you are frustrated with the enormous workload you have to bear, it's important not to let that frustration

fall onto the women you care for. They notice every facial expression, they see your eye rolls, and they hear your sighs. Please be conscious of that.

4. Most of all, remember to have empathy. Conscious maternity care means always considering how you would feel receiving the care that you are providing.

Finally, to all the mothers who have suffered birth trauma: you have a voice, and your voice matters. It is time to let your voice be heard. My heart bleeds for you, for what you have suffered and had to endure. If you are not happy with the care you received, it is important that you speak up. Write to the hospital or the manager of your maternity care provider. And if you are not happy with the response you receive, do not stop there. Find your local healthcare complaints agency and get in contact with them. Keep fighting until your voice is heard. Write, speak, scream, and demand change in maternity care. You might have already done that and felt your voice was silenced. But the voices of many cannot be silenced. Our strength is in numbers, so I plead with you to rise up, speak up, and join me in shedding light on and bringing an end to this silent epidemic of birth trauma.

If you would like to share your story of birth trauma with me, please get in touch via hello@sharonstoliar.com

Lightning Source UK Ltd.
Milton Keynes UK
UKHW020908251122
412773UK00017B/1087

9 781922 854704